Political Determinants of Health in Australia

Exposing the explicit and implicit relationships between politics, political decisions, and public policy within a planetary perspective, this book focuses on the importance of the political environment as a determinant of population health outcomes.

Political Determinants of Health in Australia brings together a team of experts in public health, health policy and planetary health in Australia to examine the political factors that determine population health outcomes. It takes a student-centred approach, explaining complex concepts in an interactive, engaging, and thought-provoking way within a logical, easy to navigate structure. Each chapter takes on key contemporary public health issues, such as family, work, diversity, housing, energy, education, food, and waste, examining it within the context of politics, policy, and health outcomes from a planetary perspective.

There is a comprehensive suite of learning activities in each chapter, catering to diverse learning styles and prior knowledge to encourage critical thinking. An essential text for students of public health, health promotion, and health policy.

Marguerite C. Sendall is an Associate Professor in the Department of Public Health, College of Health Sciences at Qatar University, Qatar, and a Visiting Fellow in the School of Public Health and Social Work at the Queensland University of Technology, Australia.

Allyson Mutch is an Associate Professor in the School of Public Health, Faculty of Medicine at the University of Queensland, Australia.

Lisa Fitzgerald is an Associate Professor in the School of Public Health, Faculty of Medicine at the University of Queensland, Australia.

T0386618

Political Determinants of Health in Australia

A Planetary Perspective

Edited by
Marguerite C. Sendall, Allyson Mutch and
Lisa Fitzgerald

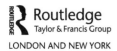
Routledge
Taylor & Francis Group

LONDON AND NEW YORK

Designed cover image: Getty

First published 2024
by Routledge
4 Park Square, Milton Park, Abingdon, Oxon OX14 4RN

and by Routledge
605 Third Avenue, New York, NY 10158

Routledge is an imprint of the Taylor & Francis Group, an informa business

British Library Cataloguing-in-Publication Data
A catalogue record for this book is available from the British Library

ISBN: 978-1-032-32533-0 (hbk)
ISBN: 978-1-032-32532-3 (pbk)
ISBN: 978-1-003-31549-0 (ebk)

DOI: 10.4324/9781003315490

Typeset in Times New Roman
by Taylor & Francis Books

Contents

List of illustrations

Figures

Table

Acknowledgements

This book was written by authors living and working in various locations across Australia on the unceded lands of Indigenous peoples. We acknowledge the ongoing efforts of First Nations (in Australia and globally) to exercise their inherent sovereignty in the good governance of their lands and the lifeforms that comprise Country, and recognise that protecting the vitality of Country is essential for addressing our planet's growing condition of environmental crisis and securing healthy futures for all life.

Contributors

Simone Bignall is a Senior Researcher in the Jumbunna Research Hub for Indigenous Nations and Collaborative Futures at the University of Technology Sydney, Australia. Drawing from her expertise as a political philosopher, she works in alliance with First Nations who are resisting settler-colonisation, exercising inherent rights to self-determination, and rebuilding collective capacities for self-governance.

Katherine Cullerton is a Senior Lecturer in the School of Public Health, Faculty of Medicine at the University of Queensland, Australia. Her research examines why evidence does not translate into policy, and how to increase the agency of advocates to better influence public health policy.

Lisa Fitzgerald is an Associate Professor in the School of Public Health, Faculty of Medicine at the University of Queensland, Australia. Lisa is a public health sociologist and qualitative researcher with research interests in the health and wellbeing of people experiencing marginalisation and the social determinants of (sexual) health.

Kerri-Anne Gill is a PhD candidate in the School of Public Health, Faculty of Medicine at the University of Queensland, Australia. Her research interest is in local food production as part of a healthy, sustainable and resilient food system and, in particular, the role of small local farms.

Jonathan Hallett is a Senior Lecturer in the School of Population Health at Curtin University, Australia. His research is based in the Collaboration for Evidence, Research and Impact in Public Health (CERIPH) and focused on health inequities and commercial determinants of health and advocacy.

Nina Lansbury is an Associate Professor in the School of Public Health, Faculty of Medicine at the University of Queensland, Australia. Her current research examines health aspects for remote Indigenous community residents on both mainland Australia and in the Torres Strait in terms of housing, water and sewerage, and women's health. She is also investigating the impacts of climate change on human health, and this involves a role as lead author on the Intergovernmental Panel on Climate Change (WG II, AR6).

Christina Malatzky is an Associate Professor in the School of Public Health and Social Work at the Queensland University of Technology, Australia. Christina principally researches relations of power and the operation of gender in the health workforce, and has particular expertise in rural studies.

Allyson Mutch is an Associate Professor in the School of Public Health, Faculty of Medicine at the University of Queensland, Australia.

Stefanie Plage is a Research Fellow at the Centre of Excellence for Children and Families over the Life Course at the School of Social Science, University of Queensland, Australia. Her expertise is in qualitative research methods, including longitudinal and visual methods. She employs these methods to contribute to the sociology of emotions, and the sociology of health and illness.

Daryle Rigney is a Ngarrindjeri Nation citizen and Professor and Director of the Indigenous Nations and Collaborative Futures Research hub in the Jumbunna Institute for Indigenous Education and Research at the University of Technology Sydney, Australia. Daryle's research and applied community practice are concerned with principles and processes of Indigenous nation-building and self-determination.

Linda A. Selvey is an Associate Professor in the School of Public Health, Faculty of Medicine at the University of Queensland, Australia. Linda is a public health physician with a background in senior levels in government and was previously CEO of Greenpeace Australia Pacific.

Marguerite C. Sendall is an Associate Professor in the Department of Public Health, College of Health Sciences at Qatar University, Qatar, and a Visiting Fellow in the School of Public Health and Social Work at the Queensland Institute of Technology, Australia. Marguerite's research is focused on health promotion settings, including workplace, education, community and health settings, employing innovative, complex and layered qualitative research methodologies to reveal more than prima facie meanings and better understand complex social and inequitable health problems in specific populations.

Rose-Marie Stambe is a postdoctoral Research Fellow at the School of Social Science and the Centre for Policy Futures in the Faculty of Humanities, Arts and Social Sciences at the University of Queensland, Australia. Rose is primarily an ethnographer whose research interests are in social and economic marginalisation and opportunities to create sustainable change.

Melissa Sweet is a public health journalist and Editor-in-Chief of Croakey Health Media, a not-for-profit public interest journalism organisation, based in Australia, with a focus on health equity and the wider determinants of health. Her work is focused on decolonising and innovation in journalism. Dr Sweet is an Adjunct Senior Lecturer in the School of Public Health at the University of Sydney.

Megan Williams is Wiradjuri through paternal family, a Professor of Public Health and a mixed-methods evaluation specialist. Megan has worked at the intersection of public health and the criminal justice system for 30 years, with a focus on prison health service delivery. Megan is Chairperson of Croakey Health Media and principal of Yulang Indigenous Evaluation.

Preface

Daryle Rigney and Simone Bignall

In the current era of late capitalism and post-imperial globalisation, planetary problems with systemic and interconnected causes threaten the health and wellbeing of all humanity. Global patterns of climate crisis, structural poverty, violent conflict and perpetual famine – resulting in processes of mass displacement and statelessness – at the same time also impact disproportionately on particularly vulnerable human populations and non-human lifeforms. The worst affected not only suffer mounting and intractable health deficits that reduce their potential for thriving; for many, their survival as such is at stake. Taking a planetary view to address such issues is both urgent and vital. It is increasingly apparent that the world's peoples need to work collaboratively to pursue the massive restructuring of social and cultural formations inherited from Western colonial capitalism, which rely on inequalities that enable the exploitative extraction of wealth and consequently tolerate the systematic production of global health disparities. It is, then, well accepted that good health is not simply a consequence of a person's robust biological constitution or lifestyle choices, but also is an outcome of beneficial social and cultural determinants. Connection to a supportive community, access to social resources, and shared participation in the intergenerational transmission of cultural practices, languages and values, all provide crucial scaffolding for healthy and happy lives. Conversely, poor health is commonly linked to negative societal influences and stressors including isolation, alienation, poverty, racism, sexism, gender-bias, domestic violence, precarious employment, excessive workloads, and chronic environmental hazards such as pollution (CSDH 2008; Fleming et al. 2019; Carson et al. 2020). Yet, to date, there has been relatively little consideration how political will, political decision-making, governance structures and political systems impact health care and health outcomes by determining the socio-cultural fabric of life. This important new book is especially significant for the direct attention it gives to the notion that health and wellbeing are significantly influenced by political factors.

Indeed, it seems strange that such factors have been so far neglected in health sector discourse. One explanation could be that international institutions concerned with planetary outlooks and the protection and advancement of human rights, such as the World Health Organization and the United Nations, have developed their programmes for action based upon a hierarchical separation between two 'generations' of rights. The Universal Declaration of Human Rights, established by the United Nations General Assembly in 1948, prioritises fundamental 'first-generation' rights that are concerned with civil and political liberties and mandate government obligations to avoid interfering in the personal or private sphere of citizens' lives. 'Second-generation' rights, then, describe the more amorphous set of basic social and economic requirements a person needs to secure their essential human dignity. They typically call for some degree of positive action on the part of governing states: to guarantee citizens access to a basic income, education, housing, health care and so forth. The right to health

DOI: 10.4324/9781003315490-1

appears in international legal instruments, including the 1946 Preamble of the World Health Organization; the 1948 Universal Declaration of Human Rights; and the 1966 International Covenant on Economic, Social and Cultural Rights. The globally dominant paradigm of Western liberalism entrenches a distinction between conceptions of 'the political' and 'the social' realms of life, with the majority designation of the right to health as a 'second-generation' socioeconomic right. This has had the effect of sidelining the ways in which health and wellbeing are directly linked to political factors.

In fact, the World Health Organization increasingly understands the social determinants of health encompass political elements at play in the 'wider set of forces and systems shaping the conditions of daily life. These forces and systems include economic policies and systems, development agendas, social norms, social policies and political systems' (WHO n.d.). Yet, this perspective also illustrates the tendency of health sector discourse to subsume political determinants within the wider category of social determinants. Accordingly, the World Health Organization observes:

> [the] unequal distribution of health-damaging experiences is not in any sense a 'natural' phenomenon but is the result of a toxic combination of poor social policies and programmes, unfair economic arrangements, and bad politics. Together, the structural determinants and conditions of daily life constitute the social determinants of health.
>
> (CSDH 2008, p. 1)

This reduction of political determinants to socio-cultural determinants is problematic because it can shift attention away from the distinctive political situations of many minority populations and how these can have systemic impacts that, in themselves, bear upon the health and wellbeing of individuals within those communities. For example, Indigenous peoples who are subject to settler-colonial domination have usually suffered the loss or reduction of their sovereignty and associated rights to self-government and self-determination; this affects the capacity of Indigenous people to enjoy the culturally safe and strong social conditions they require for their good health and wellbeing. Globally, colonisation remains a primary political consideration negatively affecting the health and wellbeing of Indigenous peoples. This highlights how the political determinants of health should not be viewed simply as elements appearing within social and cultural frames for understanding the holistic quality of wellbeing; rather, the prerequisite political status of self-governing self-determination is a foundational condition for peoples seeking to create and sustain the culturally distinctive social conditions in which their lives can flourish. Such primary political factors must therefore be addressed directly (Rigney et al. 2022).

There is strong evidence for connecting political considerations more closely with health and wellbeing programmes. One example is a recent study that shows how the lack of political self-determination can negatively impact health in the Micronesian island of Guam, which is an unincorporated territory of the United States of America. The study argues that political activism for collective self-determination can play an important role in promoting and improving health (Diaz, Ka'opua, & Nakaoka 2020). Other international studies have also found a positive correlation between collective empowerment, civil rights and increased life expectancy (Garces-Ozanne, Kalu, & Audas 2016). Furthermore, research suggests that when individual civil and political rights are enhanced, collective empowerment is also increased. This can enable communities to have a more effective political voice and advocate for better access to culturally appropriate medical services, thereby improving the health and wellbeing of both individuals and communities (Bobba 2019; Litalien 2021). Collective empowerment is particularly important for marginalised groups, as it enables them to articulate culturally specific health needs and demand appropriate services from governments. This is crucial for creating relevant and effective social and institutional frameworks that can address the health costs of societal breakdown resulting from war, colonial dispossession, and forced migration; and promote healing and reconciliation within communities (Little & Maddison 2017; Vivian & Halloran 2021).

Another reason why the political determinants of health and wellbeing have been so far neglected in health sector discourse likely concerns the way Western liberalism (and its international politico-legal frameworks) privilege a state-centric framework of 'the political'. Accordingly, governmental activity is seen to be focussed in the institutions of the sovereign state, which is considered the ultimate source of legitimate authority and jurisdiction over a society. Because health essentially refers to the 'private' realm of the body, it is conventionally understood as an area beyond or exceptional to the 'public' domain and responsibilities of the state. Clearly, there are some aspects of health and wellbeing that rely upon individuals enjoying fundamental civil and political rights to non-interference by the state in their personal lives. The control of sexuality through the criminalisation of homosexuality is an obvious case in point, having dire consequences for physical and mental health of LGBQTI+ people whose sexuality and gender identifications are disavowed as 'deviant'. In liberal societies, then, the powers of the state must not infringe upon the 'private' sphere of the individual or their family life; the duty of the state with regard to health is limited to the provision of the societal conditions required for citizens to pursue healthy lives as a matter of personal choice and self-definition. Furthermore, while some liberal democratic governments understand their public responsibilities include provision of citizen 'safety nets' such as free primary health care and a basic income, these remain issues of policy discretion dependent on citizenship status and the particular economic capacity, political will and ideological persuasion of each individual state. International principles of justice and equity, such as those enshrined in the United Nations Conventions, have no mandatory sway over these domestic matters within sovereign state jurisdiction.

Yet, in recent decades, scholars and activists alike have criticised the dominant Western liberal conception of 'the political' for its limited understanding of the scope and operation of power. Particularly as an outcome of feminist, queer, anti-racist and Indigenous struggles against patriarchal, heterosexist, racist, settler-colonial oppressions, 'the political' has increasingly become reconceived as a domain of intricate and multi-directional 'force-relations' that extend and intersect across the entire social network. Significantly influenced by anti-colonial theorists in the post-war period, by feminist assertions that 'the personal is political', and by the critique of state sovereignty led by French philosophers in the 1970s – notably including the wide-ranging scholarship of Michel Foucault – power is now often considered to operate through a wide array of social relations that bear directly, albeit often covertly, upon bodies and identities (Foucault 1980; see Bignall 2010). Rather than being the *source* of power, the liberal democratic state is then seen to be an effect or an end-point of these diffusely networked power-relations, which become institutionalised over time as they are habituated and entrenched into regular patterns of domination and social control and thereby reflected in policy-making and public discourse.

This revised conceptualisation of the scope and social operation of 'the political' in turn has implications for our emerging understandings that individual, communal and planetary health is subject to political determinants just as much as it is dependent on social and cultural conditions. Of course, it remains the case that governing states have certain responsibilities for the oversight of public health measures and the provision of primary health care services; and governmental political will, political economy, decision making, policy programmes and law clearly impact health care and health outcomes. Bearing as they do on all areas of law and policy governing how citizens' lives are lived – in their family relations, work conditions, embodied and cultural diversity, housing, energy use, environment, technology, education and agriculture – these state-controlled political determinants are the key subject matters of this book's chapters. Yet the notion that politics also concerns the social practices through which identities, subjectivities, ideologies, and cultural frameworks are formed and invested with normative powers, entails that health and wellbeing are additionally subject to political determinants wider than the powers of state. Awareness of this important point is likewise threaded throughout this book. In fact, the governing state is but one focal point (albeit a major one) for multiple sites of political action that exist within any single society. These various extra-state political agencies and authorities include, for example, the patriarchy (with feminism as a counter-authority that contests misogynist and masculinist justifications for male privilege and power); the normative institutions and cultural structures of settler-colonial Whiteness (contested by First Nations that assert their own sovereign authority in refusal of colonial domination and racial discrimination); and heterosexist religious orthodoxy (countered by queer subjectivities that assert the authority of their equal right to humanity, dignity and spirituality). Consequently, an individual's enjoyment of good health and wellbeing is not only politically determined by their ability to access crucial services provided by the state, nor solely by how well the specific needs of diverse and complex life situations are met by state policy that is required to have a general application across the entire body of the citizenry. Good health and wellbeing also are linked to the power (or capacity) of individuals, as well as the collectives they form, to exercise social agency and negotiate their positions within – and often against – the social relations in which they participate. Together, these complex operations of governmentality and agency constitute the major political determinants of health.

Understanding the political determinants of health in this way is important because it expands possibilities for orchestrating the social and cultural conditions needed for individual thriving and collective wellbeing, as well as for planetary survival. When power is not simply centred in state institutions but also extends across social networks and resides in alternative sites of authority, then political responsibility likewise is multiplied and shared amongst a great variety of non-governmental agents having capacity for socio-cultural influence and determination. Citizens, then, need not think their health provision needs are solely dependent upon the political will and good policy decisions of the governing state, although these remain significant factors in the political determination of healthy lives. Rather, individuals can look to a wider variety of powerful entities with determining agency. In some instances, such determining sources will be alternative governing bodies acting independently or alongside the formal powers of the state, such as the sovereign structures of First Nations who have assumed control of health services provision for their citizen communities. Indeed, in the settler-colonial jurisdictions of Australia, Aotearoa-New Zealand, Canada, the United States and the northern Arctic regions, mounting decades of state government policy failure correlate with the ever-deepening disadvantage of Aboriginal people; this dire situation has prompted a resurgence of First Nations governing authorities acting independently of settler-colonial state governments, intent on restoring the health and confidence of their people by self-determining the positive social conditions in which culturally distinct Indigenous communities can thrive.

Through their programmes of nation resurgence, Indigenous groups are working to rebuild their own ways of self-governance and government. This involves Indigenous nations asserting their collective identities, as polities that have persisted regardless of the harms caused by colonial invasion. Settler-colonial control, dispossession, institutionalised racism and the denial of Aboriginal sovereignties are widely discussed negative political influences affecting the health and wellbeing of Indigenous peoples. They cause well-known negative impacts, such as damage to social bonds, disruption of intergenerational knowledge transfer, and dispossession of lands and resources leading to systemic and intergenerational disadvantage. While it is important to recognise these negative impacts, it is also important to focus on positive political factors that can help Indigenous collectives exercise self-determination and improve their health and wellbeing. These positive factors include having decision-making power, being able to define and pursue goals, using Aboriginal laws to maintain order within communities, having self-governing institutions, having freedoms of political association, having independent economies and jurisdictions with decision-making powers over resources and services, and authorising access to cultural property (Fforde et al. 2020; Rigney et al. 2022). Globally, Indigenous groups are reclaiming these positive political conditions, which are crucial if First Nations are to successfully protect their environmental lands and waters from further damage. By rebuilding their cultural institutions and governance structures, First Nations are working to regain their authority and autonomy, and so to heal their societies and safeguard their Countries (see Jorgensen 2007; Cornell 2015; Hemming et al. 2019; Nikolakis et al. 2019). Thus, whereas settler-colonial governments tend to assume they are the only relevant political authority in their jurisdictions, Indigenous nation building enables Aboriginal peoples to (re) develop their capacities for sovereign self-rule. This often involves reinstating ancient institutions expressed in new forms through the creation of culturally matched governance structures that fit the current context.

Through nation rebuilding, Indigenous collectives aim to achieve effective leadership, equitable partnership, and genuine self-determination as they strive to maintain cultural, social, economic and political connections to Country and the resources necessary for supporting healthy lives, and thus sustain themselves over time. Having international relevance and application, the 'Indigenous nation building' paradigm is a theoretical and practical framework that was developed through long-term research involving Indigenous nations in the United States and Canada and further elaborated in Australia and elsewhere (Jorgensen 2007; Nikolakis et al. 2019). The research evidence shows that effective, legitimate and culturally-specific Indigenous governance is essential for the realisation of Indigenous nations' self-determined goals and ultimately, for healthy citizens and flourishing communities. Indigenous self-governance is a necessary precursor for economic prosperity and effective service delivery in policy areas including health, education, natural resource management, and housing (see Jorgensen 2007; Hemming et al. 2019; Smith et al. 2021; Rigney et al. 2022). In general, Indigenous nations progress towards their self-defined economic, health and community development goals when they exercise genuine decision-making control over their internal affairs and resources. This requires them to have effective and legitimate mechanisms of self-governance; reflect and represent the values of their citizenry; base their actions on long-term systemic strategies; and have community-spirited leadership engaged in creating positive partnerships and stable political institutions (Cornell & Kalt 2007). Indigenous nation building is a holistic framework that involves four interrelated stages: identifying politically as a cultural collective, strategising to achieve the nation's purpose, organising for self-governance, and acting sovereignly to realise collective goals (Cornell 2015). By mindfully following these steps, Indigenous nations can progress towards their self-defined economic, health, and community development goals. Often partnering strategically and effectively to maximise their capacity to reach these goals, First Nations leaders are establishing authoritative pathways towards healthier futures for their citizens (Hemming et al. 2020; Rigney et al. 2022).

When health is understood as a holistic measure of quality of life or wellbeing (which is both individual and collective, and ultimately concerns planetary environmental forces), it involves having capacity for successful integration of the full range of positive elements and relationships that constitute a healthy self. Because they are centrally about agency and capacity, health and wellbeing are also primarily about power, empowerment, and the politics of self-determination. We have indicated how Indigenous self-determination and self-governance are positive political determinants that enable the social and cultural conditions required for the good health and wellbeing of First Nations citizens and communities; and we have explained how Indigenous nation building supports these important political determinants of health and wellbeing. Nonetheless, First Nations governments with majority responsibility for the provision of health care to their citizen populations continue to face problems of inadequate funding, shortfalls in their own institutional capacity, uneven information provision and data-sharing, unequal citizen access to comprehensive health care services, and unstable political governance by nation-states in which policy frameworks continually change, depending on who has formed a government at a particular point in time. This situation frequently leads to a lack of trust that state and federal governments will not step back from their ongoing responsibilities towards First Nations as communities assume increased control over their own affairs (Rainie et al. 2015). These challenges draw our attention back to an important aspect of the idea of 'the political' as a domain of intricate and multi-directional 'force-relations' that extend and intersect across the entire social network.

According to this view of the nature and operation of power, one of the most crucial determining features of political society concerns the ways in which multiple authorities (or agencies) coexist within society and are required to relate to one another so as to negotiate their overlapping influences and perceived jurisdictions. That is, individuals and cultural communities alike do not exist in isolation but rather are relationally constituted; and these local and wider relationships are vital sites for the political determination of health and wellbeing, both for individuals and collectives. The quality of the relationship between coexisting (and sometimes competing) powers defines whether the relationship is 'toxic' or 'healthy': that is, whether it is uneven or is fairly negotiated; whether the form of interaction is unilaterally imposed by one party on another or is managed collaboratively through agreed principles of engagement. Such considerations determine the wellbeing of the participants in the relationship and also define the potential of the relationship for generating positive and healthy outcomes that can be materialised more widely or collectively (Bignall 2014; see Hemming et al. 2019). This principle of healthy co-determination applies just as much to individuals negotiating power relations in intimate settings, such as the family, as it does to First Nations governments and settler states coexisting within a political federation, such as Australia or the United States of America (Bignall 2010; Vivian et al. 2017; Hemming et al. 2019).

An important implication is that the political determination of the social and cultural conditions supporting healthy lives then significantly concerns relationship-building for positive partnerships able to influence the good governance of health. This awareness can create subtle shifts in the way power is channelled through policy planning processes. Leaders in the health sector (as is the case for other public sectors) often find themselves in the role of supplicant, advocating for the implementation of health measures at the mercy of an overriding state authority having the necessary will to prioritise public health initiatives in its budgetary decision-making. However, equipped with a sound knowledge of the relational nature of power, strategic leaders might alternatively direct their energies towards building the sectors' own centres of authority and use these to amplify key messages requiring policy attention. Ultimately, this may enable representative organisations arising from civil society to partner more effectively with the state in collaborative policy-making. The role and duties of the state would then be subtly reconfigured away from the monopoly of power and jurisdiction and towards the obligations of constructive partnership, including the enhancement of governmental facilities for listening and for coordinating the centres of authority arising from civil society.

Indeed, this kind of coordinating role is crucial for the political determination of health and wellbeing since, as this book comprehensively details, a healthy life is a multifaceted affair. Good health not only requires access to primary medical care and allied services, but also concerns identity and subjectivity; access to justice, employment and social capital; appropriate housing; well-rounded education opportunities; security of food and water; beneficial environmental conditions; agency in the context of planetary processes; and freedom from socio-cultural forces of bias and hatred such as racism and sexism. The effective political determination of health requires the coordinating input of good governance to bring these elements into balance and resonance, just as much as it needs citizens to engage actively and conscientiously in the cultivation of positive relationships that will help shape the cultural fabric of healthy societies and contribute responsibly towards the future health of the planet.

References

Bignall, S. 2010. *Postcolonial agency: Critique and constructivism*, Edinburgh: Edinburgh University Press.

Bignall, S. 2014. The collaborative struggle for excolonialism, *Journal of Settler Colonial Studies*, 4(4), 340–356.

Bobba, S. 2019. 'The central concept of empowerment in Indigenous health and wellbeing, *Australian Journal of Primary Health*, 25(5), 387–388.

Carson, B., Dunbar, T., Chenhall, R. & Bailie, R. 2020. *Social determinants of Indigenous health*. New York: Routledge.

Cornell, S. 2015. Processes of Native nationhood: The Indigenous politics of self-government, *The International Indigenous Policy Journal*, 6(4).

Cornell, S. & Kalt, J. 2007. Two approaches to the development of Native nations: One works, the other doesn't, in M. Jorgensen (ed.), *Rebuilding Native nations: Strategies for governance and development*, Tucson, AZ: University of Arizona Press, pp. 3–33.

CSDH (Commission on Social Determinants of Health). 2008. *Closing the gap in a generation: Health equity through action on the social determinants of health. Final Report of the Commission on Social Determinants of Health*, Geneva: World Health Organization.

Diaz, T., Kaʻopua, L. & Nakaoka, S. 2020. Island nation, US territory and contested space: Territorial status as a social determinant of indigenous health in Guam, *The British Journal of Social Work*, 50 (4), 1069–1088.

Fforde, C., Knapman, G. & Walsh, C. 2020. Dignified relationships: Repatriation, healing and reconciliation, in C. Fforde, H. Keeler, & T. McKeown (eds), *The Routledge companion to Indigenous repatriation: Return, reconcile, renew*, New York: Routledge, pp. 745–768.

Fleming, C., Manning, M. & Miller, A. 2019. *Routledge handbook of Indigenous wellbeing*, New York: Routledge.

Foucault, M. 1980. *Power/knowledge: Selected interviews and other writings, 1972–1977.* (ed. Colin Gordon) New York: Pantheon.

Garces-Ozanne, A., Kalu, E. & Audas, R. 2016. The effect of empowerment and self-determination on health outcomes, *Health Education & Behaviour*, 43(6), 623–631.

Hemming, S., Rigney, D., Bignall, S., Berg, S. & Rigney, G. 2019. Indigenous nation building for environmental futures: Murrundi flows through Ngarrindjeri Country, *Australasian Journal of Environmental Management*, 26(3), 216–235.

Hemming, S., Rigney, D., Sumner, M., Trevorrow, L., Rankine Jnr. L. & Wilson, C. 2020. Returning to Yarluwar-Ruwe: Repatriation as a sovereign act of healing, in C. Fforde, H. Keeler & T. McKeown (eds), *The Routledge companion to Indigenous repatriation: Return, reconcile, renew*, New York: Routledge, pp. 796–809.

Jorgensen, M. 2007. *Rebuilding Native nations*, Tucson, AZ: University of Arizona Press.

Litalien, E. 2021. Understanding the right to health in the context of collective rights to self-determination, *Bioethics*, 35(8), 725–733.

Little, A. & Maddison, S. 2017. Reconciliation, transformation, struggle: An introduction, *International Political Science Review*, 38(2), 145–154.

Nikolakis, M., Cornell, S. & Nelson, H. (eds) 2019. *Reclaiming Indigenous governance*, Tucson, AZ: University of Arizona Press.

Rainie, S., Jorgensen, M., Cornell, S. & Arsenault, J. 2015. The changing landscape of health care provision to American Indian nations, *American Indian Culture and Research Journal*, 39(1), 1–24.

Rigney, D., Bignall, S., Vivian, A. & Hemming, S. 2022. Indigenous nation building and the political determinants of health and wellbeing. Discussion paper, Melbourne: Lowitja Institute, doi:10.48455/9ace-aw24.

Smith, D., Wighton, A., Cornell, S. & Delaney, A.V. (eds) 2021. *Developing governance and governing development: International case studies of Indigenous futures*, Lanham, MD: Rowman & Littlefield.

Vivian, A. & Halloran, M. 2021. Dynamics of the policy environment and trauma in relations between Aboriginal and Torres Strait Islander peoples and the settler-colonial state, *Critical Social Policy*, 42 (4), 626–647.

Vivian, A., Jorgensen, M., Reilly, A., McMillan, M., McRae, C. & McMinn, J. 2017. Indigenous self-government in the Australian federation, *Australian Indigenous Law Review*, 20, 215–242.

WHO (World Health Organization). n.d. Social determinants of health. Available at: www.who.int (accessed 4 February 2023).

Introduction

Marguerite C. Sendall

In Australia, state governments collect taxes from people and entities and allocate these funds to resource a socially just, fair and equitable healthcare system. But is it that simple? Healthcare is much more than just a system and health is determined by more than just access to healthcare. There are clear and inseparable links between health, healthcare and politics which makes public health inherently and fundamentally political, as this quote from Baum (2015) articulates:

> Public health is a political activity because it is about change, and its history shows that public health actions are expressions of prevailing political ideologies, the beliefs of those in government and the extent to which formal power holders are influenced by interest groups.
>
> (p. 79)

Short-lived and precarious political cycles, party agendas and ideological positions, political decisions and policy agendas (e.g., food, industrial relations, trade) are critical factors that influence and determine the health of people, communities and populations (Sundin, 2019). In this way, politics is a determinant of health, directly and indirectly influencing all other determinants of health. As a new age public health student, you will practise in an increasingly complex day-to-day working environment imbued with political overtones. You will require sophisticated knowledge and advanced skills to address ever more challenging determinants of health, including the political determinants. As such, you will need the critical mind of a humanitarian, the creative mind of an entrepreneur, the communication skills of an expert writer, the passionate spirit of an artisan and the strength to argue for silenced voices. This book will help you gain a sound understanding of the complex relationship between health, healthcare and politics and how politics influences health outcomes from a planetary perspective.

This introductory chapter provides foundational knowledge about the political determinants of health and outlines the underpinning concepts required for each chapter. The first section covers the *Australian political system* acknowledging pre-colonial systems used by First Nations people and post-colonial systems embedded in British traditions, specifically the three levels of government, the Constitution and Australia's federation of states. Public policy is defined before discussing the relationship between politics, public policy and policy processes. The next section covers the *Australian healthcare system* including the international context, the World Health Organization (WHO) and Australia's role in the WHO Western Pacific Region. Australia's healthcare system will be discussed considering the three levels of administration, public and private healthcare provision and within the context of healthcare costs, the government's responsibility to provide health services and people's right to access

DOI: 10.4324/9781003315490-2

healthcare. The next section introduces the *political determinants of health* commencing with the fundamental concepts underpinning the political and all other determinants of health. Building on this, advocacy, the notion of power, political will and capital will be discussed before considering public policy, healthcare taxes and the impact of trade and globalisation. The last section introduces a *planetary perspective* which acknowledges climate change science and the unrefuted connection between human and planetary health. The term planetary health is defined before discussing the Australian and global context.

Throughout this introductory chapter, you will be asked to pause at specific junctures. **Let's think** will ask you to think about an idea in more detail by posing a question. **Let's do** will ask you to do a short activity. **Let's refresh** will ask you to refresh your knowledge about an idea. These junctures will help you think more deeply about the idea being discussed and prepare you for more complex learning activities in the following chapters.

The Australian political system

To understand the political determinants of health within the Australian context, let's begin by developing a sound understanding of the Australian political system and the policy process embedded through these systems.

Our system of government

Aboriginal and Torres Strait Islander peoples have lived on the continent of what we now know as Australia for over 60,000 years. Aboriginal and Torres Strait Islander peoples came from over 250 distinct language groups, practiced traditional land and water cultures and used sophisticated systems of law and order. After colonisation, Australia was progressively established as six separate British colonies, which came together in 1901 to form a federation governed by the Australian Constitution. The colonies handed legislative powers to the newly created parliament to form the Commonwealth of Australia, which is made up of six states and two self-governing territories, and over 500 local councils (Parliamentary Education Office, Commonwealth of Australia, 2022a).

Australia has a mixed system of government inherited from the British Westminster system. Firstly, Australia is a representative liberal democracy, one of the oldest and most stable in the world. In this democratic system, Australian citizens vote for political candidates who, as elected Members of Parliament, represent and enact laws on behalf of the constituency. Almost anywhere you live in Australia has three levels of government – the national government, the state or territory government and the local council or shire. Each level of government is elected by the people they represent (voting is compulsory in all but local council elections) and has particular responsibilities and provides certain services. The Prime Minister is Head of the national government, also referred to as the Federal or Commonwealth Government The national government has certain legislative and other powers, although some are shared with the states and territories (Parliamentary Education Office, Commonwealth of Australia, 2022a). Each state and territory government has an elected head, the Premier (or Chief Minister in the territories). States and territories have considerable autonomy because the national government does not have legal power to influence decisions (Department of Foreign Affairs and Trade, Australian Government, n.d.), although there are examples of how the Federal government has overruled decisions in the territories. Local shires and councils, known as Local Government Areas or LGAs, consist of suburbs or localities and have limited jurisdiction.

Secondly, Australia is a constitutional monarchy. Australia's head of state, His Majesty King Charles III must adhere to the Australian Constitution. Under the Constitution and on advice from the Prime Minister of Australia, the King appoints a Governor-General to act on his behalf. The Governor-General does not take part in the day-to-day running of the Australian parliament. For the most part, the Governor-General undertakes ceremonial duties but does have one extraordinary power which was executed in 1975. The Governor-General Sir Bill Kerr sacked the Prime Minister, Gough Whitlam. This event has gone down in Australian political folk lore with much debate.

Let's do

You should read about Whitlam's social reform agenda and what led to his sacking. This podcast recounts the event: https://www.abc.net.au/radio/programs/the-eleventh. You can find Whitlam's speech, in response to his sacking, here: https://www.youtube.com/watch?v=CZGE4tVdsOk. Reflecting on what you have read and heard, what might social health, the healthcare system and Australia look like today, if Whitlam had not been sacked?

Australia is governed by a set of rules outlined in the Australian Constitution. The Constitution outlines how federal and state parliaments make laws about national matters, for example, trade, foreign affairs, immigration and defence (Parliamentary Education Office, Commonwealth of Australia, 2022a). In particular, the Constitution explains how the Parliament (local representatives), the Executive (the government) and the Judiciary (the courts) share power to make and manage laws. Known as the separation of powers, this arrangement ensures each group has their own area of responsibility and no group has all the power. Essentially, the Parliament makes and changes the law, the Executive enacts the law, and the Judiciary settles legal disputes (Parliamentary Education Office, Commonwealth of Australia, 2022b). In 2023, the Albanese Labor Government proposed a constitutional amendment to enshrine an Indigenous Voice to Parliament. The Indigenous Voice to Parliament would consult with Aboriginal and Torres Strait Islander peoples tasked to advise the Australian Parliament and Executive about Indigenous affairs. Referendums are required to change the Constitution. Voting in a referendum is compulsory and success requires a double majority – 50% of the national majority and a majority of voters in four of the six states.

Let's think

This referendum states: 'A proposed law: To alter the Constitution to recognise the First Peoples of Australia by establishing an Aboriginal and Torres Strait Islander Voice.' What are the proponents' and opponents' arguments about the proposed alteration to the Constitution?

Our public policy process

By now you've heard the term 'policy' more than a few times, and no doubt you've also heard it discussed by politicians and the media – it is a term frequently used during election campaigns with much fanfare and debate. So, what is policy? Buse, Mays and Walt (2012) define policy as a: 'Broad statement of goals, objectives and means that create the framework for activity. Often takes the form of explicit written documents but may also be implicit and unwritten' (p. 5). Public policy, which includes policy for health, is the process of decision-making within governments (Palmer & Short, 2014). Public policy involves many different types of statements, intentions and actions and can involve direct and indirect legal and regulatory action. These activities are undertaken and enacted by elected politicians and government policymakers on behalf of the public to deal with specific matters of public importance. Policymakers are guided by stages of development known as the 'policy' cycle which starts with an agenda, moves to formulation and legitimation, then implementation and finishes with evaluation (Palmer & Short, 2014).

Despite the clear pathway outlined in the policy cycle, policy is not 'neat and tidy'. Policy can be dull and straightforward and rarely involves transparent processes. It may involve struggles between competing interests – some may be highly visible while others are conducted quietly on the sidelines or behind closed doors. These competing interests (sometimes called policy actors, stakeholders or vested interests) make policy important and provide insight into the political determinants of health. Public policy and politics are closely intertwined because political ideology, expertise and authority shape all policy. Despite frequent political inertia, parliamentarians are positioned to drive healthcare policy change and enact legislation. Unsurprisingly, Russell, Lawrence, Cullerton and Baker (2020) found parliamentarians reflect their political party's ideology and therefore shape public health policy responses aligned with those views. For example, Green parliamentarians reveal the Party's core value of social justice through systemic government intervention. Liberal parliamentarians reveal the party's core values of liberalism and neoliberalism through advocating more personal responsibility and less government regulation. Labor parliamentarians are somewhere in the middle but are often aligned with social liberalism which promotes universalism including healthcare, for example, Medicare and the redistribution of resources.

So how does a health issue get onto the policy agenda? This is a critical question, the focus of much literature and central to our discussion about the political determinants of health. Policy decisions are influenced by a range of factors including public opinion, media coverage, the nature and complexity of the issue and the ideology of decision makers – and not necessarily the best scientific evidence. Influenced by these factors, politicians have the power to implement (or not) policies which impact population health outcomes. This results in a policy decision-making process which is complex and contextually embedded and where policy makers often act on values-based considerations rather than evidence.

Let's think

What is your knowledge or experience of policymaking in the current social, political, and economic environment?

Many countries have experienced a proliferation of neoliberal policies over recent decades but what does neoliberalism mean? Neoliberalism is a political ideology, sometimes described as a broad policy model or agenda, which emerged in the late 1970s and 1980s grounded in the work of Milton Friedman (Barnett & Bagshaw, 2020). The USA and the UK conservative governments (Thatcher in the UK and Reagan in the US) led the development and implementation of neoliberalist agendas adopting policies which promoted and prioritised markets, privatisation and competition, individualism and freedom of 'choice', small government and deregulation. These policies impact the social determinants of health, for example, junk-food marketing which influences childhood obesity and health and economic burden. Such priorities continue to shape state operations and direct policy decisions around the world, including Australia. Within neoliberalism, health is treated as a commodity, an economic good, which subsequently impacts how health is measured and determines who is responsible for managing health (individuals) and the provision of healthcare (how healthcare is provided and by whom). Under neoliberalism, the *commercial determinants of health* are enacted as private providers use market power to access resources and influence policy decisions. The focus on individual responsibility for maintaining and managing health corresponds with the emphasis on addressing the health behaviours of individuals and re-directs the focus away from the socially embedded nature of health, health practices and the *social determinants of health* (Viens, 2019).

Multisectoral healthcare is well understood as an approach to better health outcomes. However, the realisation of multisectoral healthcare policy to address health inequities and better health outcomes has been sluggish and patchy. Baum and Friel (2017) note most evidence is at a technical level, for example, health inequity facts. The authors suggest there is a poor theoretical and practical understanding of the environment for effective policymaking and a much better understanding of the political and healthcare policy processes is required. To this end, vigorous enquiry about political and healthcare policy processes is required to address the determinants of health. This lack of progress can be attributed to complex healthcare policy systems which fail the policy coherence test. That is, healthcare policy goals and actions fail to achieve a synergy across multiple sectors. This is most obvious in the UN 2030 Agenda for Sustainable Development. Many UN Sustainable Development Goals (SDGs), such as poverty, gender equality, water and sanitation, impact local and global health inequities. Achieving effective and sustainable action and outcomes to improve daily living conditions which affect health, for example, urban planning and quality schooling is still difficult. Even more difficult is action for politically delicate matters such as trade, taxation and racism, which challenge existing influential norms and assumptions of power.

The Australian healthcare system

Now you have learnt about the Australian political system, let's look at the Australian healthcare system. This will build your foundational knowledge to better understand and critique complex concepts associated with the political determinants of health from a local and global perspective.

Our global health environment

Over the last 20 years or so, the term global health has gained international visibility due to media and public interest and as an emergent research priority. Global health addresses the determinants and inequalities in power, resources and governance, is universal and rights based, is locally connected and conceptually political and influenced by privatisation, biomedical and technocratic reductionism and the inherited authority of the Global North, that is, high-income countries such as the USA, the UK and Europe.

Let's think

What do you understand by the term, 'the Global North'? You should also read about the Global South.

Recent international events like Black Lives Matter, gun violence and police brutality shone a light on healthcare policy and healthcare deficits around the world, including Australia. Ironically, the COVID-19 pandemic showed the world that governments *can* mobilise and respond in a timely way, for example, the increased use of green space and digital technologies in the pandemic.

Australia's healthcare system is situated within and influenced by global health, and other environments. Seminal public health documents such as Canada's Lalonde Report (1974) and the Ottawa Charter for Health Promotion (1986) have influenced government healthcare policy, practice, and the healthcare system to some degree. However, the true extent of real and potential influence has not been realised mostly because there is a significant time lag between global documents and, if any, recognition and shift in healthcare policy in Australia. This lag is often further detained by the politicisation of the health priority.

Let's think

Think of a current example of a global health issue which has shaped health policy here in Australia. Then think of a current example yet to be adopted into Australian healthcare policy and the reasons why this has not happened.

Established in 1948, the World Health Organization (WHO) is an independent agency of the United Nations auspiced with authority to direct and co-ordinate public health, including health emergencies and access to healthcare, at global, regional and country levels. More than 7000 staff worldwide collaborate with the governments of 194 Member States and other stakeholders to achieve the WHO founding vision; *to ensure the highest attainable level of health for all people*. WHO helps its member countries to, for example, build strong national healthcare systems, in disaster preparedness and address Non-Communicable Diseases (NCDs). The WHO works alongside the UN Security Council (UNSC) which deals with threats and risks to international peace and security through a health security lens.

As an active Member State, Australia has worked closely with the WHO for nearly 70 years. Australia is part of the WHO Western Pacific Region. The Western Pacific Region supports Member States to achieve better health outcomes across 37 countries and areas and nearly 1.9 billion people. Like many countries in this region, Australia shares health challenges such as the ageing population, the rising burden of NCD's and a finite and receding healthcare budget. Together, the WHO and Australia have worked collaboratively on strategies to address global health priority issues at a regional level. Examples of political alliances and working together in the region include the eradication of smallpox, and aid for the victims of Cyclone Winston (2016) in Fiji and the Christchurch earthquake (2011) in New Zealand.

Our local health environment

The Australian healthcare system is administered at three levels of government, which have been described earlier. The Federal government sets the national healthcare agenda (national goals and targets, health priority areas), establishes auspicing bodies and collects taxes to fund the healthcare system, for example, Medicare. The Federal government allocates funds to state and territory governments to administer hospitals and acute care services. State governments are responsible for non-acute services such as school health and Public Health Units which manage, for example, meningococcal outbreaks. Local governments oversee environmental health which includes the monitoring, surveillance, and prevention of infection. This varies across jurisdictions as some states and territories have a broader public health mandate.

Since the early 1970s, public health in Australia has been grounded in the principles of social justice and driven by a strong labor movement. As part of a broader social reform agenda, a publicly funded, universal healthcare insurance scheme, including the Pharmaceutical Benefits Scheme and Medibank, now Medicare, was introduced. Australia also has a private healthcare system which assumes those who can afford to pay, have the right to quicker access to healthcare services and reduces the demand for public healthcare. The Australian healthcare system has a unique feature, the relationship between public and private healthcare. Australians are encouraged to purchase private health insurance through federal government tax incentives. Australians are charged a 2% Medicare levy. Those who purchase private health insurance can claim a 1% Medicare rebate in their annual tax return. However, fewer Australians are purchasing private health insurance, especially young adults who identify perceived value and trust in insurers as barriers (Tam, Tyquin, Mehta & Larkin, 2021).

Let's do

Why do you think this is? Make a list of pros and cons for buying private health insurance.

Governments have a specific role in healthcare through policy and funding and a broader role in the economy, environment, culture and society. Underpinned by philosophical and social ideologies, governments implement healthcare policies which impact people's behaviours to achieve desired healthcare outcomes. In Australia, as in other countries, the government must strive to balance the responsibility to improve population health with individual rights. This balance of responsibility and rights is reflected in political party ideology.

Let's refresh

Remember, we touched on neoliberal policy in the previous section. To better understand this concept, please read this journal article by Russell, Lawrence, Cullerton and Baker (2020) about how public health nutrition, in particular, junk-food marketing to children is politically constructed. You can find the citation in the References.

Legislation, education and other policy options, such as environmental change, welfare policy, budget allocations, research funding and taxation, are a continuum of intervention to escalate social and behavioural change. However, all options to accelerate these changes are responsive to social and cultural tolerance.

Let's think

Let's consider these political determinants of health – seatbelt legislation, lockdowns in the COVID-19 pandemic, childhood immunisation, alcohol regulation and urban design. For each example, you should think about how the social and behavioural change happened and how the population tolerated these interventions. What are some other examples?

Governments should consider healthcare policy change by taking account of existing and dynamic social contexts. For example, tobacco legislation across Australia was well tolerated and moved quickly because social norms had already changed. In states like Queensland, the population had adjusted its behaviour to comply with a smoke-free environment before legislation. As more and more restrictive legislation was enacted and implemented, there was little resistance because the population had already responded. There have been many memorable anti-smoking campaigns.

Let's refresh

You may remember this Queensland campaign, 'No-one smokes here any more', which symbolises the success of tobacco legislation in Australia: https://www.youtube.com/watch?v=qe4GqUFVuVk.

There is an interdependent and complex relationship between economic development, growth and prosperity and the growth of humans, communities, populations and societies. As healthcare costs rise in high-income countries like Australia, there are diminishing returns on investment because the health dollar is spent according to cost benefit and cost-effectiveness ratios which favour treatment over prevention. Public health has strong arguments for good returns on spent health dollars and advances gained over the long term. Tobacco smoking is a good example – federal and state governments have implemented a broad spectrum of policies to reduce tobacco smoking over the last 40 years demonstrating a decrease in the health impacts of smoking. However, long-term gains are politically problematic because vote-winning is linked to funding support for short-term healthcare outcomes, such as the reduction of waiting lists for elective surgery.

Let's think

How do you think public health can better market long-term gains to the voting public and politicians?

The political determinants of health

Now you have a sound understanding of the Australian political system and the Australian healthcare system, let's introduce the concept of the political determinants of health. To help situate the political determinants of health, you will start by revisiting health determinants more broadly, followed by a discussion about the politics of health.

Our health determinants

There is overwhelming empirical evidence for the relationship between everyday living conditions and health outcomes. This relationship is known as the social determinants of health – the conditions in which people are born, grow, live, work, and age that impact physical and mental health outcomes. These social determinants include many factors, for example, a sense of control over one's life, social support and exclusion and living and working conditions. The social determinants of health also include structural factors embedded in the socioeconomic-political context, and broader economic, social and cultural processes. These structural factors produce and distribute systems of power and generate inequities between groups embedded in institutionalised forms of racism, sexism, gender-bias, classism, and ageism (Solar & Irwin 2010). In particular, institutional racism characterises the discrepancy in the social determinants of health because it influences social, cultural and economic conditions and environments laden with unequal generation and distribution of power. Furthermore, the narrative about the determinants of health and health inequities is underpinned by the commercialisation of health as a commodity and stereotyping of people's socioeconomic status.

Let's think

In this conversation, is there an 'elephant in the room'? That is, are there classist structures hidden in Australian society?

There are other determinants of health, for example, the commercial determinants or the strategies and approaches used by the private sector to maximise power and profits through the promotion of products which impact health outcomes. The other key determinant, the focus of this book, is the political determinants of health. There are direct and indirect links between politics, healthcare policy and health outcomes. The political determinants of health, such as power and control, governance and resource distribution, systems and decision-making, and inequities and empowerment, are the political structures, processes and decisions which impact health outcomes (Sendall, 2022). These ideas are explicitly highlighted in seminal public health documents such as the Lalonde Report (1974), the Declaration of Alma-Ata (1978) and the Ottawa Charter (1986). Despite these global mandates, the political system in Australia, including the actions of federal politicians and the policies of political parties, have shaped the determinants of health.

There is a slowly increasing narrative, and maybe awareness of, the political determinants of health.

Let's refresh

Think back to the example of junk-food marketing to children highlighted in the previous section.

Policing is another example. Policing harms vulnerable populations through a legacy of racism, prejudiced power and criminalisation and disciplinary reactions to social problems.

Let's do

Discuss this idea with your family and friends to better understand others' views about policing and its impact on health outcomes.

More broadly, the neoliberal politics adopted by governments accentuate the political determinants of health. Neoliberalism has three main strategies: (1) competitive markets; (2) private markets; and (3) deregulation to encourage freedom of 'choice' and benefit the economy and frugal expenditure on health and social services. In New Zealand, these strategies have negatively impacted the population's health. For example, children, people from low socioeconomic backgrounds and Māori and Pacific islanders have unduly assumed the burden of income inequality driven by privatisation and competition and the unequal distribution of the 'determinants of health' (Barnett & Bagshaw, 2020). Neoliberalism in New Zealand has abated to some degree but there should be a focus on 'upstream' healthcare initiatives and more social investment where benefits outweigh costs and ensure social and cultural equity goals are reached.

Our health politics

Public health practitioners who work fervently at the local and community level are, by the nature of their work, advocates. Advocacy is a core competency for public health practitioners.

Let's refresh

Revisit your understanding of advocacy.

Advocacy is underpinned by ethical principles and entrenched in the concepts of social justice. Advocacy is about people's rights, freedoms and liberties, the distribution of power and population inequality. Advocacy strives for social or collective good and to influence public policy to improve health outcomes in populations who have less control and power over their lives. Advocacy is a ground-up process driven by community connectedness and social capacity building which empowers communities and populations to engage with the political process. These local coalitions and alliances can influence broader societal reform by mobilising sentiment and progressing the agenda. New technologies such as social media platforms can help galvanise this collective power of populations with shared beliefs and values.

Let's think

Do you think advocacy should be more politically and morally overt for any real change to occur?

By its very nature, advocacy is political because it challenges those who hold power. Power is inherent in the healthcare policy process because the policy process represents the distribution of power in society. This power imbalance starts from the beginning of the healthcare policy cycle (is the problem on the agenda?) and continues throughout policy formation, implementation and evaluation (Baum & Friel, 2017). Politicians, policymakers, commercial and business entities, and community groups with different and conflicting agendas hold differential power to influence decisions.

There are three other important and intertwined concepts underpinning the political determinants of health. The first concept relates to power. Friel et al. (2021) argue an understanding of the distribution and use of power is critical to our understanding of the political determinants. They identified three categories of power: (1) agentic power wielded by individuals and individual organisations; (2) structural power embedded in the rules, norms and mandates of institutions and systems; and (3) discursive power, which exists within deeper ideas and discourses, and through policy decisions. The second concept is political will. The concept of political will links to public health advocacy because it aligns with the underpinning public health ideologies of social justice and human rights. The idea of 'political' is embedded in public health, it can inform political action and inaction and drive political will (Galea & Vaughan, 2019). Political will is complicated by political cycles and political success. Consequently, advocacy should be underpinned by a deep understanding of how politics work. Only then, will public health be entrenched in the political psyche. Ineffective systematic action by governments, despite evidence on the social determinants of health, is often blamed on a lack of political will. Little is known about the effectiveness of advocacy in the creation of political will and the role it plays in the development and adoption of policy supporting health equity (Baum et al., 2020). Public health, tasked to address human and ecological health, should be cognisant of politics and its own political nature and should build political credentials to maintain pressure for change. Essentially, there is a critical need to engage in the political process and influence decisions which shape healthcare policy. The third concept underpinning the political determinants of health is political capital. There are many examples of political capital. Essentially, political capital is the ability to influence political decisions, benefit from accumulated power based on trusted relationships and good will, and influence the process of politics, policymakers, politicians and political parties. Political capital is saved, spent wisely or not, lost and gained and can mobilise advocates and activists, populations, other politicians and parties to achieve the desired outcomes.

Let's think

Think back to Gough Whitlam's speech after he was sacked by the Governor-General in 1975. Can you think of a contemporary example of political capital?

Some public policies are coercive, that is, they infringe on people's civil liberties and rights by restricting behaviour, for example, seatbelt legislation. In more detail, let's consider if restricting people's behaviour for better health outcomes offsets small limitations on the freedom of individual choice. Some experts claim governments should use coercive policy as a lever to modify environments and influence the population's behaviour because it can be very effective, for example, a tax excise on alcohol. Others argue from a civil-rights perspective, that people should be free to decide for themselves.

Let's think

Do you think people should be free to choose, for example, to wear a seatbelt or stop at a red traffic light?

Taxes on health can be beneficial for public health, for example, tobacco taxes are designed to reduce the rates of smoking and improve health outcomes. Jain, Baker and Chalkidou (2020) acknowledge the cost effectiveness of healthcare taxes in producing income to address population health outcomes. However, their use is limited because due process and execution are not applied to tax decisions as in other healthcare interventions. Complicating national healthcare policy further is the impact of trade and globalisation, for example, international trade rules and the influence of global entities with varying interests and authority. Vigorous governance ensures trade policy considers health, social justice and sustainability to mitigate health risks and maximise health benefits. Newly created trade governance arrangements because of Brexit (the UK's departure from the EU) provide a context to explore the relationship between governance and health and social justice. van Schalkwyk, Barlow, Siles-Brügge et al. (2021) found failings in the four governance pillars of the UK trade policy. The UK government failed to respond to overwhelming evidence about the impacts of trade policy on healthcare and equity and strong systems of governance.

Let's think

This study was undertaken in the UK. Do you think the findings about international trade are relevant in Australia, in the region and globally?

A planetary perspective

Finally, you will position your understanding of the political determinants of health within a planetary perspective. To do this, let's consider important concepts associated with the climate and the planet's health by considering human health. Now, you are well versed in the foundational knowledge required to develop an in-depth understanding of the political determinants of health in the following chapters.

Our planet's climate

The science is conclusive – the world's environment is changing. Climate change is real and happening now, but these changes are more than just climate. From the contamination of water, soil and air and the degradation of marine systems, unprecedented rain and drought events, rising sea levels and melting polar ice caps, record-breaking heatwaves, the extinction of species due to a lack of arable land, and changing land use to food production using half the planet's habitable surface. Experts from a range of backgrounds agree it is imperative to take climate action now to stop, or at least slow down, climate change before the effects intensify and the damage is irreparable.

In Australia, public sentiment has shifted and health, corporate and other sector leaders are driving change. Successive reports have contributed to this shift. For example, the State of the Climate report released by the Bureau of Meteorology and the Commonwealth Scientific and Industrial Research Organisation (November, 2020) report warming across the Australia is now up to 1.44 (0.24) – 8°C since 1910. Similarly, the recent Royal Commission into National Natural Disaster Arrangements explicitly recognises climate change has increased the risk and impact of bushfires. Teal Independents have changed the political landscape and re-energised the debate on climate change legislation in Australia. For example, Independent MP Zali Steggall, backed by the Australian Medical Association and major businesses, introduced the Climate Change (National Framework for Adaptation and Mitigation) Bill 2020 into the Federal parliament. There is broad recognition of the need for climate action, for example, to progressively move away from fossil fuels and invest in renewable energies. This shift will benefit the natural environment, secure energy supplies, and open up new prospects for the employment sector.

Despite this shift in sentiment, climate action in Australia, as in many other countries, is political. In 2016, Australia signed the Paris Agreement on climate change. Under this non-binding Agreement, Australia was required to submit enhanced nationally determined contributions to end climate change by 2020. The UK and the EU agreed and China committed to net zero carbon emissions by 2060. However, the Australian government has not agreed to net zero carbon emissions by 2050. Experts propose the Australian Government should agree to a 50% reduction in carbon emissions by 2030 to impact global warming.

Let's think

Why do you think Australia is reluctant to commit to the targets set by the Paris Agreement? Think about your answer from a political perspective.

Experts such as Tait (2022), suggest an accurate political-economic diagnosis of our unwell planet can be attributed to the behaviour of large corporations and governments regulatory failure. The 'corporatocracy' has shifted the political system from 'the public good' to winning office. Parliamentarians are caught up in a corrupt system of, for example, buying influence to win a seat. Political leaders bend to corporate needs rather than science unless it suits them otherwise, and corporate-driven decisions are bereft of community benefit, for example, progressing climate action. Climate action should include risk reduction measures, including housing, transport, and urban and rural planning policy and ambitious all-sector carbon emissions targets. The Australian healthcare sector is not a major carbon emitter in comparison to, for example, the energy, mining and agricultural sectors. Nonetheless, the sector should lead by committing to net zero carbon emissions by 2040, in line with the National Health Service in the UK, preferably with the states and territories responsible for implementing evidence-based interventions.

Our planet's health

There is a well-recognised and inextricable link between human health and the planet's health. Human health and planetary health are symbiotic, they depend on each other. Human health has improved overtime. Humans are living longer and better, in less poverty and in better economic circumstances. However, progress in human health has shown little respect for natural resources, many non-renewable, and has outpaced sustainable regeneration. Conversely, the planet is at risk because of the rapid and expedient degradation of the natural environment (United Nations Climate Change, n.d.). The UN Environment Program's most recent report (February 2021) states: 'Humanity's environmental challenges have grown in number and severity … and now represent a planetary emergency.' Ironically, this new era in the Earth's geology, the Anthropocene, distinguished by humans' extraordinary effect on the planet's natural condition puts gains in human health at risk by destroying the very thing which keeps humans alive (Planetary Health Alliance, 2023). The progressive development of a sophisticated and responsive civilisation depends on the health of humans, and humans judicial care for thriving natural ecosystems.

The term planetary health is a reasonably new concept in public health discourse.

Let's think

What do you think the term 'planetary health' means?

Often misunderstood as climate change, planetary health is a transdisciplinary social movement, focused on understanding humans' impact on earth's natural systems and finding solutions for human and the planet's health (Planetary Health Alliance, 2023). Broadly, the discipline of planetary health is a shared, co-operative alliance concerned with the interaction and relationship between people and environments or, more specifically, human health and the health of the natural environment in which humans live and depend. Supporting this movement is The Lancet Countdown, an independent surveillance programme to monitor the health profile and impact of climate change (Watts, Amann, Arnell, Ayeb-Karlsson et al., 2021). This international collaboration includes leading academic organisations and UN agencies drawing on a wide range of expertise including climate, social, political and data scientists, engineers, energy, food and transport experts and public health professionals.

Conclusion

In this introduction, you have learnt about the underpinning concepts and fundamental ideas of the political determinants of health in Australia. Now, you have a better understanding of the Australian political system, the Australian healthcare system and the determinants of health from a planetary perspective. These foundational concepts will help you understand the complex relationship between each of these ideas, how they influence each other, to what extent, what are the likely unmitigated scenarios for human and planetary health in the future and how you, as individuals, practitioners, advocates, professional associations and activists might interrupt dire outcomes. Throughout the next chapters, you will develop a more sophisticated, contextualised and nuanced grasp of political and public health, and the political determinants of health. This newfound knowledge will help you develop the skills you will need to navigate the complexities of futuristic practice.

References

Barnett, P., & Bagshaw, P. (2020). Neoliberalism: What it is, how it affects health and what to do about it. *The New Zealand Medical Journal*, 133(1512), 76–84.

Baum, F. (2015). *The new public health* (4th edn.). South Melbourne, Victoria: Oxford University Press.

Baum, F., & Friel, S. (2017). Politics, policies and processes: A multidisciplinary and multi-methods research programme on policies on the social determinants of health inequity in Australia. *BMJ Open*, 7(12), e017772. https://doi.org/10.1136/bmjopen-2017-017772.

Baum, F., Townsend, B., Fisher, M., Browne-Yung, K., Freeman, T., Ziersch, A., Harris, P., & Friel, S. (2020). Creating political will for action on health equity: Practical lessons for public health policy actors. *International Journal of Health Policy Management, 11*(7), 947–960. https://doi:10.34172/ijhpm.2020.233.

Buse, K., Mays, N., & Walt, G. (2012). *Making health policy: Understanding public health* (2nd ed.). Maidenhead: McGraw-Hill Education.

Department of Foreign Affairs and Trade. Australian Government. (n.d.). Introduction to Australia and its system of government. Available at: https://www.dfat.gov.au/about-us/publications/corporate/proto col-guidelines/1-introduction-to-australia-and-its-system-of-government (accessed 9 January 2023).

Galea, S., & Vaughan, R. D. (2019). Public health, politics, and the creation of meaning: A public health of consequence. *American Journal of Public Health*, 109(7), 966–968. https://doi.org/10.2105/AJPH.2019.305128.

Jain, V., Baker, P., & Chalkidou, K. (2020). Harnessing the power of health taxes. *BMJ*, 369: m1436. https://doi:10.1136/bmj.m1436.

Palmer, G., & Short, S. (2014). *Health care and public policy: An Australian analysis*. South Yarra, Victoria: Palgrave Macmillan.

Parliamentary Education Office. Commonwealth of Australia. (2022a). Australian system of government. Available at: https://peo.gov.au/understand-our-parliament/how-parliament-works/system-of-governm ent/australian-system-of-government/ (accessed 9 January 2023).

Parliamentary Education Office. Commonwealth of Australia. (2022b). Introducing … Australia's system of government. Available at: https//peo.gov.au/understand-our-parliament/how-parliament-works/system-of-government/introducing-system-of-government/ (accessed 9 January 2023).

Planetary Health Alliance. (2023). Planetary health. Available at: https://www.planetaryhealthalliance.org/planetary-health (accessed 9 January 2023).

Russell, C., Lawrence, M., Cullerton, K., & Baker, P. (2020). The political construction of public health nutrition problems: A framing analysis of parliamentary debates on junk-food marketing to children in Australia. *Public Health Nutrition*, 23(11), 2041–2052. https://doi:10.1017/S1368980019003628.

Sendall, M. C. (2022). Political determinants of public health. In P. Liamputtong (ed.), *Public health: Local and global perspectives* (3rd ed.). Cambridge: Cambridge University Press.

Solar, O., & Irwin, A. (2010). A conceptual framework for action on the social determinants of health. Geneva: WHO Document Production Services.

Sundin, J. (2019). Public health is politics. *Interchange, 50*, 129–136. https://doi.org/10.1007/s10780-019-09367-z.

Tait, P. W. (2022). Good governance for planetary and the public's health: A 21st century agenda for supporting and re-energising the public's health. *Australian and New Zealand Journal of Public Health, 46*(2), 101–104. https://doi:10.1111/1753-6405.13209.

Tam, L., Tyquin, E., Mehta, A., & Larkin, I. (2021). Determinants of attitude and intention towards private health insurance: A comparison of insured and uninsured young adults in Australia. *BMC Health Services Research*, 21(1), 246. https://doi:10.1186/s12913-021-06249-y.

United Nations Climate Change. (n.d.). Planetary health. Available at: https://unfccc.int/climate-action/un-global-climate-action-awards/planetary-health (accessed 9 January 2023).

van Schalkwyk, M. C. I., Barlow, P., Siles-Brügge, G., *et al.* (2021). Brexit and trade policy: An analysis of the governance of UK trade policy and what it means for health and social justice. *Global Health, 17*(61). https://doi.org/10.1186/s12992-021-00697-1.

Viens, A. M. (2019). Neo-liberalism, austerity and the political determinants of health. *Health Care Analysis*, 27, 147–152. https://doi.org/10.1007/s10728-019-00377-7.

Watts, N., Amann, M., Arnell, N., Ayeb-Karlsson, S., et al. (2021). The 2020 report of The Lancet Countdown on health and climate change: Responding to converging crises. *Lancet*, 397, 129–170. https://doi:10.1016/S0140-6736(20)32290-X.

Part I
Political Determinants of Our Selves

1 Family and Work

Christina Malatzky

> To liberate society from gender- and class-inequality would be a transformation that is almost beyond the bounds of imagination … It is … essential that the whole balance between work and non-work life should be re-thought …
>
> (Oakley, 1980, pp. 299–300)

Learning objectives

After studying this chapter, you should be able to:

1 Understand how politics affects the health of families, the effects of politics on work cultures, and the role of state and government in these processes.
2 Analyse the interconnections between gender equality, the creation of inclusive, sustainable work futures, public health, and planetary health.
3 Assess how effectively policies target the drivers of social and economic inequalities to protect and promote the health and wellbeing of families and women.
4 Critique the success of contemporary policy initiatives in fostering systemic recognition of and assigning value to unpaid care work by promoting the equitable distribution of this work.

Snapshot: Giving it all – in a burning world

In a world governed by neoliberal logic, families have been left relatively on their own to manage the very real health, economic, and social consequences of climate change and the COVID-19 pandemic. Neoliberalism skilfully deflects structural responsibility onto the individual. It erases social inequalities as non-issues, mere products of individual 'choices', whilst being an economic system fundamentally sustained by this relation (Malatzky, 2013). Women are undeniably at the centre of families and family politics. The social role of raising children and providing (unpaid) care to the family is assigned to women who participate in the paid economy. Women are giving it all – to their families, workplaces, and communities – and are often disproportionally affected, in a range of ways, by the implications of declining planetary health. This underscores how gender equality and creating inclusive, decent work sit at the heart of environmental, economic, and social justice agendas. As this chapter highlights, simultaneously transforming gender and power relations in the domains of the family and work, whilst, as Ann Oakley (1980, p. 299) suggested, 'beyond the bounds of imagination', is essential to the restructuring of human life needed for a better future.

DOI: 10.4324/9781003315490-4

Let's begin

This chapter focuses on the interconnections between gender (in)equality, (un)sustainable futures, and public and planetary health. Research and socio-political commentary from Australia and elsewhere are drawn on to analyse and critique the nature and effects of politics and the resulting policy environment for various public health issues situated within the family and work domains. The chapter begins with an analysis of how children and young people – disproportionally affected by climate change – are positioned within political discourse pertaining to climate action. The ways children and young people use their power to counter government inaction are highlighted. In the context of increased competition for resources related to environmental degradation, the focus moves to how politics, as the exercise of power, positions and affects women's lives and intersects with public health and sustainable development. An analysis of gender-based violence (GBV) is presented as a case example, where, again, there have been comparably weak political leadership and policy responses. Examining these intersections illustrates the co-dependency of human and planetary health and, thus, of environmental justice and feminist agendas centred on social justice and gender equality. This section ends by putting these analyses into a broader context and discussing the changing nature of family formations and the political conditions in which families are situated.

Centring the health impacts of politics and policy in the work domain, the focus turns to contemporary debates about safety at work and the public health issue of sexual harassment, a form of GBV. This examination focuses on the types of politics that create workplace environments in Australia where sexual harassment is enabled, the limitations of current policy responses, the contributions of the #MeToo movement to gender justice, and the move towards decent work futures. The related issue of the right to equal opportunity is then explored through an analysis of paid parental leave policies. This analysis draws out the connections between the aims of these policies and gender equality and the need for the redistribution of work within Australia to develop more sustainable and just ways of living in the future. With this goal in mind, the chapter ends with an important discussion about the care economy and, in the context of an ageing population, questions how the care of older Australians will be enabled through policy instruments that address the disproportionate health effects of care work borne by women.

The health impacts of politics and policy on our family

Children and young people

Many far-ranging political and policy-related issues are relevant to children's and young people's health in the contemporary world. However, it is difficult to conceive of a single more pressing implication of politics and policy for children and young people than the unfolding climate emergency. The wide-ranging environmental changes occurring because of a changing climate, including rising global temperatures and sea levels and extreme changes in weather-related patterns causing increased incidences of events like flooding and drought, are already directly affecting living conditions in many parts of the world. Countries in the Global South, which, ironically, have contributed least to the greenhouse gas emissions driving climate change, are currently among the most affected (Singh et al., 2022). However, given the interconnections at a bio-environmental level through the globe's climate system and the biosphere, and at a socioeconomic level through the intensification of globalisation, nowhere on Earth will escape the effects of climate change.

There is little doubt that in the medium – and certainly the long – term, today's children and young people will face the brunt of climate change and its flow-on effects; they will inhabit a fundamentally altered world to the one into which they were born. Even now, children and young people are particularly vulnerable to and disproportionally impacted by climate change. Almost half the world's children currently live in countries deemed at 'extremely high risk' of the effects of climate change (UNICEF, 2022, para. 3). According to the United Nations Department of Economic and Social Affairs (2019), approximately 85% of the world's young people live in the Global South, where extreme weather events like drought and floods are currently concentrated. These more frequent events cause widespread displacement and increase food insecurity. Climate change has thus been identified as a key determinant for child health directly and indirectly linked to patterns in childhood morbidity and mortality.

Children and young people in what are currently high-income economy countries will not escape the consequences of climate change. For example, recent climate modelling predicts that children in Australia today will experience four times as many heatwaves, three times as many droughts, and 1.5 times as many bushfires and floods compared to previous generations (Save the Children, 2021). Relatedly, Singh et al. (2022, p. 1) describe the 'public mental health crisis' caused by climate change, or more accurately, the political inaction in response to climate change, within these contexts in which children and young people are particularly affected. These researchers argue for greater engagement in and advocacy from the medical community around the injustices of climate change for young people and the importance of protecting children's rights to a safe and secure future. Others have also documented the emotional burden experienced by children and young people as a consequence of climate change and the growing uncertainty about what the future holds in the context of ongoing political apathy amongst many of the world's most influential leaders. Governments can reduce the extremes of climate change, assist in the transition to more sustainable energy sources, and support the health and wellbeing of future generations if they act now. Children and young people in many parts of the world have expressed frustration and anger about the decision of many political leaders, especially those of wealthy countries in the Global North, to effectively not act – to prioritise 'economic growth' and short-term political gains over planetary health. The most extensive survey on climate anxiety administered to young people globally in 2021 found that the majority feel betrayed and abandoned by governments that they see as failing to adequately respond to climate change (Hickman et al., 2021).

Children and young people have not been passive in the face of rising global inequalities and uncertainties created by climate change and the COVID-19 pandemic. Young people have launched legal cases and formed political parties to hold current governments to account for protecting them from climate change. They have written action plans for other young people and youth organisations to operationalise their fight to address climate change and its health effects. There has been a burgeoning of youth-initiated and led social and protest movements such as the UK Uncut movement and, in Spain, the Indignados movement. Globally, young people are drawing critical attention to the trajectories current political leaders have plotted for their citizens through movements such as School Strike 4 Climate and Fridays for the Future and proposing alternative futures made possible by different ways of living (Hayward, 2021). These movements are underpinned by the social values of 'ecological care, compassion, intergenerational justice and social responsibility' that directly challenge those of conservative politics and the far right (Hayward, 2021, p. 1).

Indeed, some conservative politicians have sought to characterise the leadership demonstrated by young people as naïve and dismiss and marginalise the arguments and interests of children and young people within public debates (Hayward, 2021). For example, when many young Australians protested about the government's inaction on climate change in 2018, then Prime Minister Scott Morrison's response was to tell them, and the school system, to be 'less activist' and to 'go to school'. In 2019, Morrison told young Australians, 'don't worry, be happy', and stated that he wanted:

> children growing up in Australia to feel positive about their future, and I think it is important we give them that confidence that they will not only have a wonderful country and pristine environment to live in, that they will also have an economy to live in as well. I don't want our children to have anxieties about these issues.
>
> (Parkinson, 2019)

Rather than including young people – as the world's most impacted citizens – many governments have excluded them from the political discussion and decision-making processes. Some international entities, such as UNICEF, are attempting to shift these responses and encourage governments to develop what they refer to as child-sensitive climate and environmental policies that centre children and young people's particular vulnerabilities to climate change *and* their influential role in climate action. Young activists are also promoting human rights-based approaches to climate change that seek to empower young people in the domains of policy-making, governance, and global investments in climate change.

Let's do

Drawing on documentation from UNICEF and Australian government websites, review how well Australia is tracking with developing child-sensitive climate and environmental policies. Consider the case examples profiled by UNICEF and formulate a short briefing paper that argues for one key policy that would improve Australia's commitment to Action for Climate Empowerment.

Let's think

Have you or any of your family and friends been engaged in protect movements? How did you or your family and friends take part and why did you think it was important to be involved? Consider ideological positions.

Spotlight: Advocacy action

Health professionals, especially medical doctors, remain influential actors in contemporary societies and their participation in advocacy for climate action is recognised as critical to building political will. Emergency physician Kimberly Humphrey's article, 'Climate Action – It Is Up to You' (Humphrey, n.d.), for *onthewards*, a community of junior doctors committed to 'empowering the next generation of patient-centred doctors' argues that young doctors can be particularly persuasive in climate action discussions. Humphrey offers the following ideas for health professionals wanting to advocate for climate action:

- Join organisations that are active in the climate advocacy space and can 'elevate your voice' (para. 9) and provide opportunities to influence policy.
- Take up writing and speaking opportunities at whatever level; talking at a local primary school can be impactful – it doesn't have to be the United Nations.
- Undertake training in advocacy, media and lobbying.
- Meet and lobby politicians of all levels: local, state and federal.

Women

In conceptualising politics as the exercise of power through which people are governed in a diversity of ways, it is clear that women and people identifying as and with diverse genders and sexualities have been subjects of, subjected to, and agents in health affecting political struggles historically and in the contemporary context. Various issues could be focused upon, from sexual and reproductive health to cancer prevention and screening, body image, lifecycle changes and ageing, and homelessness. However, here the persistent issue of GBV has been selected as a salient example of how the politics of gender intersect with public health and the future of sustainable development. Drawing on understandings derived from the United Nations and scholarly literature, van Daalen et al. (2022, p. e505) define GBV as 'violence directed towards a person because of their gender or violence that affects persons of particular genders disproportionately due to structural and societal power imbalances', which is inclusive of interpersonal/intimate partner violence, domestic violence, family violence, and physical, emotional, sexual, and technological forms of violence, as well as slavery practices like human trafficking. At the root of GBV is enduring gender inequality, the ongoing social acceptability of narrowly defined concepts of masculinity and femininity, and the so-called traditional gender roles these endorse (van Daalen et al., 2022). Indeed, in studies seeking to identify the predictors of violence-supporting attitudes, low levels of support for gender equality were identified as the strongest (Phillips et al., 2015).

During the COVID-19 pandemic and the resulting increased competition for limited resources, rates of GBV accelerated worldwide. This is consistent with current evidence that GBV increases during natural and human-instigated crises and disasters (van Daalen et al., 2022). The International Union for Conservation of Nature (2020, para. 2) found that GBV is commonly used to (re)assert privileges and control over resources and maintain existing power relations that underpin gender inequality 'to the detriment of livelihoods, human rights, conservation and sustainable development'. Women and girls actively advocating for sustainable development in the context of environmental degradation are especially targeted. These patterns illustrate the interconnectedness between human and planetary health, environmental justice, and feminist agendas. Gender equality is a central goal in planetary health and responses to climate change, given the short- and long-term consequences of issues like GBV (van Daalen et al., 2022).

It is potentially easy or politically convenient for those in positions of privilege and influence to position GBV as predominantly an issue for 'elsewhere' in public discourse – usually, the Global South, where examples of what constitutes this kind of violence may be more visible or readily identifiable. However, GBV remains the most common form of violence in highly wealthy Western industrialised countries in, or considered part of, the Global North and has been labelled the silent epidemic (Phillips et al., 2015). In Australia, for example, an average of one woman per week is murdered by a current or former partner, 1 in 3 women have experienced physical violence, and 1 in 5 sexual violence before the age of 15 years (Our Watch, 2018). Despite its prevalence and the well-documented evidence of far-ranging and serious consequences for the physical, mental, social, and emotional health and wellbeing of women, gender and sexually diverse people, and often children, many incidences of GBV go unreported. This is in part because those who experience GBV fear they will not be believed or protected from the perpetrator(s). The dominant ways in which GBV is spoken about and popularly understood that often trivialise experiences of GBV demonstrate the legitimacy of these fears and ultimately undermine calls for substantial political action in this field (Phillips et al., 2015).

Limelight

In attempts to shift dominant discourses about GBV, there has been considerable feminist advocacy around the need for strong policy and resourcing to protect and support those experiencing GBV. Several high-profile cases, such as the brutal murder of 11-year-old Luke by his father in front of his mother, Rose Batty, during a cricket practice session, in 2014 and the murders of Hannah Clarke and her three children, aged 6, 4, and 3, who were doused in petrol and burnt alive in a car by her husband and the children's father in 2020, have also drawn the experiences and consequences of GBV most acutely into the public domain. This has resulted in the introduction of new laws around coercive control – defined as a 'pattern of assault, threats, intimidation, humiliation, and other abuse that erodes a person's autonomy and ability to flourish' – in the Australian state of Queensland, where such behaviour is now a criminal offence.

Mainstream media has played a key role in drawing horrifying examples of GBV into the public consciousness but has been selective in whose stories are given coverage. The horrendous treatment of First Nations Australian women, who are murdered at up to 12 times the national average, often fails to attract the same degree of intense coverage. For example, it would be relatively safe to claim that the majority of people in Australia know the name Hannah Clarke; however, it would be far less safe to claim the majority would know the name R. Rubuntja, a prominent anti-domestic violence community campaigner who was murdered – deliberately hit by a car and reversed over multiple times, causing catastrophic and ultimately fatal injuries – by her then partner. It is important to be critical about whose experiences of GBV are centred in the public domain – not to dismiss the worthiness or legitimacy of those whose are, but to consider the intersections between the politics of representation, gender, and other powerful forms of inequality also rooted in inequitable power relations. This is also relevant in the context of framings within policy. For example, heteronormativity remains the assumed norm, and fixed gender concepts continue to be uncritically adopted in policy.

Spotlight: Power dynamics

In their article 'Violence Regimes: A Useful Concept for Social Politics, Social Analysis, and Social Theory', Jeff Hearn, Sofia Strid, Anne Laure Humbert, and Dag Balkmar (2022) explore the utility of 'violence regimes' as a concept for informing politics and policy pertaining to forms of violence, including GBV and environmental violence. Violence regimes are defined as 'the governance and production of forms and aspects of violence' (p. 566). The article centres analytical attention on different types of violence and how violence is 'a cause and con-sequence of social realities' – that is, of politics, policy, and policy development (p. 568). As an analytical tool for policy, violence regimes make plain how different kinds of violence are interconnected and highlight the tendency of policy responses to violence to ignore these interconnections; violence policy remains, in the norm, fragmented, with different types of violence dealt with in different domains and at different levels of government, underpinned by different understandings of what constitutes violence and how violence can be measured. The concept of violence regimes assists with expanding political understandings of the nature and breadth of violence – and thus, understandings of the range of policies that address the interconnections of types of violence needed to shift cultural norms.

Global context

An issues paper on the criminalisation of coercive control released by the Australian Women Against Violence Alliance (2021) contextualises Australia's legislative landscape and the sub-sequent (lack of) uptake pertaining to coercive control compared to other countries. In Australia, there remain inconsistent definitions and understandings of GBV amongst policymakers and the wider community, and differing views on how coercive control should be addressed through policy across the states and territories. By 2021, only one state in Australia had criminalised non-physical forms of GBV – Tasmania – where the maximum sentence was two years. In contrast, coercive control was criminalised across England and Wales in 2015, Scotland in 2018, and Ireland in 2019. Implementing such legislation has been particularly successful in Scotland, where many police officers have been trained and cases and convictions are recor-ded, with the offence carrying a maximum sentence of 14 years. A key point of distinction in the lead-up to and consequent uptake of coercive control legislation between parts of Australia and Scotland is the extensive nature of community consultation and awareness raising about the nature and harms of coercive control. From an Australian feminist perspective, it is critical that a nationwide understanding of GBV is developed so that a whole-of-system approach to addres-sing GBV can be taken. To achieve this, resourcing to engage the community and train key actors in the system to respond to the needs of victims/survivors is essential.

Family

Hayes and Higgins (2014) argue that families are the most complex foci for policy and pol-icymakers because they manifest both private and public concerns. Weston and Qu (2014, p. 17) characterise families as 'the most basic unit of society in which much "caring and shar-ing"' occurs and most children are raised. Families have a critical role in protecting and pro-moting the health and wellbeing of human populations across global societies. Bogenschneider (2014) explains that family policies are those that explicitly aim to 'support' or regulate the primary functions of families. These include how families are formed and potentially dissolve or change over time through procreation and social practices like marriage and divorce and the adoption of children, the nature of partner or intimate relationships, and how the financial, economic and, to some degree, social needs of family members are addressed by the state. In this context, many family functions have remained relatively stable over time (Hayes & Hig-gins, 2014). However, other policies (e.g., those on broader social concerns, such as housing, unemployment, and poverty) implicitly affect families. Consequently, Bogenschneider (2014) explains how the effects of these broader policies should be assessed through a family lens. This argument is made in the context of the recognised interconnections between the state of families and the broader communities and societies they are part of (Hayes & Higgins, 2014). With these interconnections in mind, Bogenschneider (2014) stresses the importance of considering how families work in ways that support broader units of society and society as a whole and how policies support families' functions.

It is in this context that much family scholarship challenges the perception that families are largely static, unchanging social units and articulates how family formations change in often complex ways in response to changing social conditions (Hayes & Higgins, 2014) that over time stimulate policy reform. For example, in many Western industrialised countries, changes in the socio-cultural norms related to the status and rights of women induced changes to legislation regulating marriage and divorce (Weston & Qu, 2014). In these contexts, marriage rates have been declining, and divorce and cohabitation rates have been rising for some time (Weston & Qu, 2014). Many family scholars view the current degree of change and fluidity within families as unprecedented (Sassler & Lichter, 2020). What have, in the past, been understood as alternative or marginal family forms are now growing and have implications for contemporary policy. In this context, Weston and Qu (2014) describe the increasing numbers of same-sex couple families and grandparent families wherein grandparents care for and cohabitate with dependent and non-dependent grandchildren without the children's parents. There has also been a rise in separated couple families with children taking on 'equal' caring responsibilities, which is a strong preference among today's young people (Sassler & Lichter, 2020). However, single-parent families remain most likely to be living in poverty. Further, contemporary family literature documents a rise in couples 'living apart together' (LAT), which reflects socio-political change and has policy implications. Sassler and Lichter (2020) argue that contemporary gender and race relations, the politics of class, and economic and related health inequalities are crucial to explaining these changing patterns in family formation. Family forms are essentially adaptations to broader relations of power embedded within social processes of globalisation, including economic restructuring and health inequalities. This supports Bogenschneider's (2014) argument that policies targeting the drivers of these broader societal processes – and the social and health inequalities (re)produced – are central instruments affecting families. In a world infected by COVID-19 and experiencing irreversible climate changes, the need to rapidly change policies intending to support – and those affecting – contemporary families remains pressing.

Indigenous perspective

A Lowitja Institute (2022) discussion paper, 'Indigenous Nation Building and the Political Determinants of Health and Wellbeing', authored by Daryle Rigney and colleagues, provides an Indigenous Australian perspective on the impacts of politics and policy for Indigenous families and what is needed to secure the future wellbeing of Indigenous communities. Emphasis is given to the critical importance of sincerely recognising, at all levels of government and the broader community, the ongoing impacts of past colonial policies that removed Indigenous children from their families and communities. Given the violence and brutality inflicted upon Indigenous Australian families through this and other policies, it should be no surprise that the ability to self-govern child protection and child health are key priorities for First Nation communities across Australia. Here, nation building, defined as 'a process Indigenous political collectives can follow to enhance their own foundational capacity for self-rule and self-governance' (p. 8), is critical to enabling Indigenous governing bodies to enact the rights of their citizens who are also, simultaneously, subject to regimes of colonial power. The authors of this discussion paper articulate the critical role of nation building in responding to family violence issues and in assisting children and young people to 're-possess' their land by facilitating connection to Country, which is central to the health and wellbeing of Indigenous families.

The health impacts of politics and policy on our work

Safety at work

Sexual harassment is a key issue when it comes to safety in contemporary workplaces. It is a form of GBV and is defined as unwanted or unwelcome sex-related behaviour at work that the recipient experiences as offensive, intimidating, hostile, degrading, humiliating, and a threat to wellbeing (Huseth-Zosel et al., 2021). As seen in the case of other forms of GBV, sexual harassment is predominantly experienced by women across the lifespan and by sexual minorities (Huseth-Zosel et al., 2021; O'Neil et al., 2018). Patriarchal power structures that enable and support misogynist attitudes, male entitlement, adherence to rigid gender norms, and processes that subjugate and objectify women in broader society make the kinds of workplace environments in which sexual harassment is not only possible but frequently cemented into organisational cultural norms (McDonald, 2020). According to O'Neil et al. (2018) in *The Lancet*, in Australia, around 40–60% of women have been sexually harassed in their workplace. In European countries like Finland, women are twice as likely to experience GBV at work than men. The impacts of sexual harassment on physical, psychological, emotional, social, and occupational health are borne mainly by women. The development of negative perceptions of self-worth (Jagsi, 2018) and psychological conditions, including depression, anxiety, and post-traumatic stress disorder, which are well-established risk factors for chronic disease, are known health consequences of sexual harassment, as are damaging changes to blood pressure and heart rate and the numerous flow-on consequences of stress (e.g., increased use of alcohol and cigarettes; O'Neil et al., 2018). It is important to note that these health consequences have been documented amongst those who have been sexually harassed themselves and those who have witnessed or know someone who has been sexually harassed and become exaggerated when sexual harassment is not treated seriously within the workplace (Huseth-Zosel et al., 2021; O'Neil et al., 2018). From an organisational and broader societal perspective, the consequences of sexual harassment and the flow-on effects for workplace cultures include a significant loss of productivity, avoidable turnover and absenteeism, and the associated under-utilisation of the population's skills, expertise and knowledge, and unrealised human potential (O'Neil et al., 2018). Consequently, sexual harassment in the workplace is a major public health issue that raises important social and ethical questions about global work futures and the challenges we face in creating safe, healthy and sustainable work environments.

Goncharenko (2022) emphasises that social movements poignantly reflect and shape community perceptions of issues that require serious scrutiny and reflection from the public. The now well-known hashtag MeToo was originally used by New York-based community organiser Tarana Burke in a grassroots campaign to engage underprivileged girls experiencing sexual abuse (Goncharenko, 2022; McDonald, 2020). In 2017, #MeToo was used by several women to share their experiences of sexual harassment by then Hollywood producer Harvey Weinstein on social media platforms (Goncharenko, 2022; McDonald, 2020). #MeToo quickly trended and developed into a global social movement aimed at raising awareness about the serious consequences and prolific nature of sexual harassment in the workplace (McDonald, 2020) and how women who report sexual harassment are routinely marginalised, stigmatised, and subjected to retaliation (Jagsi, 2018). The #MeToo movement challenged the predominant framing of sexual harassment as a personal matter, where shame is operationalised as a mechanism to control and silence those adversely affected. The movement also clearly delineated sexual harassment as a serious and pervasive act of criminal violence in the public consciousness. It has also led to critical, collective reflections on, as Goncharenko (2022, p. 16) articulates, 'the relationship between the abuse of power and accountability' and has spearheaded growing demands for much greater organisational accountability, something that many sectors remain hesitant to accept. In this context, the #MeToo movement has been a powerful platform to advocate for systemic action that shifts current workplace norms that enable, perpetuate, and effectively silence the realities of sexual misconduct (McDonald, 2020).

The #MeToo movement has increased public awareness about the kinds of societal and organisational conditions that enable and perpetuate sexual harassment. In her analysis of what the #MeToo movement has achieved, McDonald (2020) specifies that these conditions include the intertwining of authoritarian hierarchies and patronage systems into the fabric of the workplace that creates a dependency on senior, often male, colleagues for training and career advancement opportunities. McDonald (2020, p. 2) also outlines the established evidence that sexual harassment is more likely to occur in the workplaces of conventionally masculinised occupations where conservative gender norms dominate: sporting codes in which 'celebrity status and entitlement lead to a lack of accountability for one's actions' and often, excessive use of drugs and alcohol; organisations where 'strong male bonding [and] codes of mateship and loyalty … intensify sexism and encourage group loyalties to override personal integrity'; and industries that 'haze' and 'initiate' newcomers using abusive means.

Despite increased awareness and understanding of the issue, McDonald (2020) and others such as Huseth-Zosel et al. (2021) argue that the #MeToo movement has not resulted in the systemic change necessary to disrupt the bedrock of sexual harassment. Gender inequalities and the patriarchal power structures that maintain these imbalances persist, and many of the regulatory systems that contribute to the perpetuation of sexual harassment are unchanged. For example, in Australia, GBV is still not recognised as an occupational hazard, which keeps the onus on individuals to make formal complaints using their workplaces' internal reporting processes (McDonald, 2020). It is well documented that these processes are ultimately designed to protect the organisation (Jagsi, 2018) and do not require workplaces to make structural changes to address the root causes of GBV (McDonald, 2020). This provides the context for why it has been necessary for the #MeToo movement to evolve into the Time's Up initiative, which raises funds for those who have been sexually harassed in their workplaces to take legal action (Goncharenko, 2022).

Similar to other feminist interventions, whilst creating a vector for potentially inclusive and transformative dialogue amongst those who have been sexually harassed in their workplaces (Huseth-Zosel et al., 2021), the #MeToo movement has also provoked considerable backlash, which has health implications in and of itself (O'Neil et al., 2018). Examples of how the backlash has manifested include the labelling of initiatives designed to respond to workplace sexual harassment as 'anti-men' and levelling of the powerful construct of 'merit' at these same initiatives to suggest that efforts to redress gender inequality unfairly advantage women based on gender rather than their ability to do the job (McDonald, 2020). Using these techniques again diverts organisational accountability for enduring gender inequalities that have a variety of consequences for safety at work. While providing a vehicle through which women have been able to 'go public' and share the realities of sexual harassment, social media is not unproblematic for feminist politics. For example, McDonald (2020, p. 3) highlights how social media 'allows men to watch, search for and intervene in feminist conversations, derailing and redirecting their focus'. Further, as discussed earlier in reference to the representation of GBV and constructions of legitimacy and worthiness around whose stories are told and through what frame, other forms of social inequality and discrimination influence whose stories of sexual harassment are taken up in social media and whose accounts are believed (McDonald, 2020).

Let's do

In pairs or small groups, discuss how categorising GBV as an occupational hazard could challenge the patriarchal power structures that enable sexual harassment in your workplace.

Indigenous perspective

Indigenous Australians have identified cultural safety in the workplace as a critical aspect of work safety. Cultural safety has been defined as: 'the recognition that one needs to be aware of and challenge unequal power relations at the level of individual, family, community, and society. In a culturally safe environment, each person feels that their unique cultural background is respected, and they are free to be themselves without being judged, put on the spot, or asked to speak for all members of their group' (Cull et al., 2018). Contemporary workplaces have a social responsibility and, in the case of public service, a legislative requirement to create a culturally safe environment for workers and clients/patients/consumers/users (State of Victoria, 2021).

Spotlight: Advocacy action

Public health and other professionals can advocate for improving the cultural safety of workplaces by:

- Promoting and genuinely engaging in training and professional development, especially opportunities that focus on understanding one's own cultural location and perspective, unpacking how the power of Whiteness operates in the workplace, and taking responsibility for addressing unconscious bias, racism and discrimination (Wilson, 2011).
- Developing an understanding of diversity within and across Indigenous communities and cultural systems.
- Contributing to discourse and dialogue about ongoing processes of colonisation, Indigenous empowerment and sovereignty, dominant culture, Whiteness, and fear about working in this space.
- Advocating for genuine cross-cultural collaborations and partnerships.

Equal opportunity

Equal opportunity – the right of every person to participate freely and equally in all areas of public life, including the workplace (State Government of Victoria, 2019) – benefits individuals, families, communities, and broader society socially and economically. Research has demonstrated that women's increased participation and opportunities for career advancement in the paid labour market are critical to the UN's Sustainable Development Goals (SDGs) of achieving gender equality and the empowerment of women and girls and promoting sustained, inclusive and sustainable economic growth, full productive employment and decent work for all (Raub & Heymann, 2021), which are preconditioned on a healthy planet. Fostering equal opportunity is a central objective of many governments. People's access to opportunities that promote and protect good health (e.g., decent, secure income) can be effectively influenced through policy (Raub & Heymann, 2021). Many countries have passed statutory laws and developed progressive social policies that seek to address systemic discrimination based on gender and other social identifiers that remain a powerful barrier to equal opportunity. Social policies that aim to foster equal opportunity in the workplace have broader effects for gender and other forms of (in)equality and the equitable distribution and accessibility of the social and material resources needed to produce sustainable, healthy societies.

Paid parental leave – paid leave for parents after the birth and, in some jurisdictions, the adoption of a child – is a key policy instrument in many national strategies for fostering equal opportunity. In all OECD countries except the United States, paid parental leave is a statutory right (Raub & Heymann, 2021). Paid parental leave policies have been described as a core plank in the social protection floor:

> [the] sets of basic social security guarantees that should ensure, as a minimum that, over the life cycle, all in need have access to essential health care and basic income security which together secure effective access to goods and services defined as necessary at the national level.
>
> (International Labour Organization, 2022, para. 1)

They are instrumental for the specified target to 'recognize and value unpaid care and domestic work through the provision of public services, infrastructure and social protection policies and the promotion of shared responsibility within the household and the family' (Sustainable Development Solutions Network, 2012, Section 5.4) in achieving the SDG of gender equality and the empowerment of women and girls (Raub & Heymann, 2021). The evidence is well-established that paid parental leave directly benefits families' health and women's labour market outcomes (OECD, 2017; Raub & Heymann, 2021). Likewise, the role of paid parental leave in promoting gender equality is well documented. What is also established in the literature, but less pronounced in public discourse, is the importance of men taking paid parental leave for the health of the whole family unit (OECD, 2017) and critically, 'dis-establishing' rigid gendered ideas about the division of labour (Margaria, 2021; Raub & Heymann, 2021).

Men who take paid parental leave are more likely to take on an equitable share of unpaid domestic and child-caring work with their partners, which positively affects the health of women, children, and men (OECD, 2017). In countries where a higher proportion of men take paid parental leave and there are increased childcare subsidies, women's participation and progression within the labour market improves (Margaria, 2021). Encouraging men to take parental leave may also help to address the gendered discrimination women of childbearing age experience in the workplace, such as not being employed in the first place, being kept on short-term contracts with little job security, or being passed over for promotion in this life stage (OECD, 2017), by shifting gendered assumptions around who cares for children (Malatzky, 2013). It is currently uncommon for men to take substantial parental leave (OECD, 2017). To improve the rates of men taking parental leave, some countries offer men 'strong incentives', restructuring paid parental leave policies to include the concept of shared parental leave and non-transferrable leave entitlements, and creating separate policies for paternity leave (Margaria, 2021). These policy adjustments are informed by an understanding of the gender relations and norms that maintain the assumption that women are the primary carers of small children – a societal-level barrier men encounter when taking on caring responsibilities (Margaria, 2021). It has been argued that this level of understanding is critical to the effective design of paid parental leave schemes.

Let's refresh

There are 17 SDGs with 169 targets that collectively represent a 'plan of action for people, planet and prosperity' that 'seeks to strengthen universal peace' and requires all countries and stakeholders to act in collaborative partnership to implement (United Nations Department of Economic and Social Affairs, 2019). In 2015, all UN Member States adopted this plan and recognised the interconnected nature of its goals. The UN publishes an annual report on how the implementation of the plan is progressing throughout the world, which includes a range of relevant data. Workplaces within the UN Member States have an important role to play in implementing and making progress towards the SDGs. Review the UN SDGs via the UN website and your workplace's strategic plan and/or KPIs (you can refer to your university's strategic plan if needed). Consider how the SDGs are reflected (or not) within this plan and/or KPIs. Share your conclusions with your tutorial group. To extend this work, break into small groups and select one of the group's workplaces as a case study. Develop a proposal for a new initiative that could be introduced in this workplace that would simultaneously progress the organisation's strategic plan and the SDGs.

Global context

At the time of publication, Australia's publicly funded national paid parental leave scheme, legislated in 2010, provides a primary carer of a newborn or adopted child with a right to a wage at the federal minimum rate for a maximum of 18 weeks in the first year following the birth or placement of the child while they are on leave from paid work (Malatzky, 2013). The scheme is available to those with an individual annual income of AUD150,000 or less who have worked at least one day a week for at least 10 of the 13 months preceding the birth/ adoption (Buckmaster, 2022). A separate scheme that provides two weeks, again at minimum wage, was introduced for fathers in 2013.

Despite being a signatory to the same international human rights instruments as other OECD countries (e.g., the International Labour Organization, which influences the formation of social policy; Lynn, 2018), Australia's parental leave scheme does not compare well on the global stage. Australia was the second last OECD country to introduce a publicly funded parental leave scheme, with the United States still to act. Unlike elsewhere, Australia's scheme is taxable, has no superannuation contributions, and offers a minimum rather than a replacement wage (Malatzky,

2013; Lynn, 2018; Buckmaster, 2022). All these features have drawn criticism, as have the restriction requirements on time worked to be eligible for the scheme, which disadvantages those in insecure work – mostly women – and the overall positioning of the scheme as essentially a form of welfare as opposed to a workplace entitlement, which it is in most other OECD countries (Lynn, 2018). While poor across the board, the uptake among fathers has been particularly poor in Australia compared to other OECD countries (Lynn, 2018). Schemes in Scandinavia, often touted as the global leader in this space, are considerably more generous, as is the German scheme. In France, the Netherlands, and Eastern Europe, where there is a greater political appetite to do more to facilitate uptake among men, wages are largely, and in some cases entirely, replaced, and paid parental leave policies are just one strategy in a suite of policy responses to the changing gendered nature of the workforce and broader gender relations. Publicly funded childcare, for example, features strongly in these other settings.

In comparison, in Australia, there is a question as to how well the scheme is targeting gender inequality, and, despite some proposed amendments, reforming the current scheme has not been a political priority (Buckmaster, 2022). Critically, the Australian scheme is not accompanied by a progressive childcare policy. Childcare remains one of the most significant costs for Australian families with young children, to the extent that, for many, the amount of money earned by returning to paid employment after the birth/adoption of a child could be substantially consumed by childcare fees (Hurley et al., 2022).

Let's do

You are a senior policy advisor in the Australian Federal Government's Department of Social Services. The Social Services Minister has asked your team to provide some advice on potential strategies for facilitating or enabling a greater proportion of men to take parental leave. Hold a thinktank with your team in which options can be proposed, discussed, and debated. Then, select the solutions most likely to be effective in the Australian context and prepare a short presentation for the Minister.

Caring duties

Unpaid care and domestic work undertaken by families in homes and the broader community is commonly referred to as the care economy (Power, 2020), which encompasses the substantive proportion of care work in contemporary societies. Using the most modest of estimates, unpaid carers are collectively at least twice the size of the formal care workforce (Ferrant et al., 2014). This labour is of crucial societal and economic benefit (Cylus et al., 2019). Whilst caring duties are commonly discussed in reference to those involved with raising children, the focus of these discussions must be broadened in political and public health circles.

Globally, populations are ageing, and more people are living with disability for more years than in the past (Brimblecombe, Pickard, et al., 2018). The need for care is rising. These changing demographic profiles are occurring in the context of broader social change affecting the formations and dynamics within families. For example, in many Western industrialised countries, fewer families live in intergenerational households (where grandparents live in the same home as their children and grandchildren) than in the past. It is now also more common in couple families for both partners to be engaged in paid work. This invariably changes the possibilities available to families when it comes to caring for older family members and creates further complexities for negotiating unpaid care work with paid work, the structure of which has been slow to evolve with the changing needs and contexts of families (Malatzky, 2013). However, it is important to be critical of how, in much of the literature, this is framed as a consequence of women's increased participation in the paid workforce. Such framings implicitly reflect, but uncritically, the highly gendered nature of care work. Women undertake most unpaid care work in the world, doing anywhere between two and 10 times more unpaid care work than men – on average, 75% of unpaid care and domestic work in families and communities (Ferrant et al., 2014; Power, 2020). Power (2020) draws attention to how the COVID-19 pandemic has dramatically increased this already disproportionate allocation of care work in women's lives. Without state intervention, it will have ongoing effects for years to come. In this context, Power (2020) underscores how the care economy is sometimes referred to as the hypocrisy economy, as women undertake paid work in addition to shouldering the lion's share of unpaid care work.

As discussed earlier, in outlining how achieving gender equality and empowering all women and girls can be achieved, the United Nations specifies the need for unpaid care and domestic work to be recognised and valued 'through the provision of public services, infrastructure and social protection policies, and the promotion of shared responsibility within the household and the family' (Sustainable Development Solutions Network, 2012, Section 5.4). Therefore, recognising unpaid care work is a critical social, economic, and equity issue for the sustainability of contemporary societies (Brimblecombe, Pickard, et al., 2018). It is imperative that current state supports, including policies, and the promotion of these are considered through a gender equity lens and deliberatively 'encourage or enable' men to take on more caring duties (Power, 2020, p. 67) rather than implicitly assuming it is women for whom these supports are relevant. Policymakers need to actively consider ways to break this assumption. As Ferrant et al. (2014) argue, the central activity of caring needs to be re-distributed between genders, families, and the state. There is currently a long way to go before this objective is achieved.

Given the current global economic system in which most nation-states are embedded, a significant area of focus for policymakers has been on how those who provide unpaid care can be best supported to remain employed in paid work – how to support carers to balance their caring responsibilities with those of paid employment. This is in response to recurrent findings that being responsible for providing unpaid care to family members – a responsibility still predominantly assigned to women – often leads carers to reduce their paid working hours, take on less well paid work, or leave paid work altogether, which has detrimental effects for the wellbeing of individuals and families in the context of rising poverty, and carries a substantial cost to society (Brimblecombe, Fernandez et al., 2018). The consequences of unpaid care work on carers' physical and mental health and wellbeing have also been well documented in the literature (Brimblecombe, Fernandez et al., 2018) and, given the gendered nature of unpaid care work, are disproportionately affecting women.

The corresponding types of support legislated by states have included schemes that provide financial and psychological support, respite care and training, and legal entitlements such as leave provisions and flexible work arrangements for carers (Brimblecombe, Fernandez et al., 2018). The provision of high-quality, fit-for-purpose social care services has also been identified in contemporary research as a critical means of supporting unpaid carers to remain employed. How these services have not only not attracted increased funding but have been incrementally eroded in many wealthy countries is of deep concern to communities and has drawn substantial critique from socially engaged researchers and social policy experts. So too have the ongoing implications of these funding conditions for local governments and the community sector; in many places in the world, they are key providers of support and services to older people and carers (Brimblecombe, Fernandez et al., 2018).

In developing social and economic supports for families in the context of an ageing population, as Cylus et al. (2019) suggest, potentially harmful and misleading assumptions must not drive political discussions and potential public health responses. For example, the assumption that people necessarily become 'dependent' and are thus a 'burden' on society once they reach a pre-defined age and the related misperception that older people do not continue to make a substantial economic and social contribution to broader society. Older people are also most often the providers as well as the recipients of unpaid care work. Thus, initiatives designed to support older people's health and activity levels have an important role within a suite of well-considered responses to supporting older people, families, and communities (Cylus et al., 2019). As discussed earlier in this chapter, how policies are designed is crucial. In this space, policies must be carefully crafted to redress the effects of entrenched gender norms and stereotypes (Ferrant et al., 2014) and ageism. On this point, we must consider ways to reduce the costs associated with an ageing population that enhance (rather than ignore) older people's contributions to family life and broader society (Cylus et al., 2019).

Spotlight: Policy process

In their article, 'Tapping the Sustainable Development Goals for Progressive Gender Equity and Equality policy?', Gabriele Koehler highlights how: policymakers face immense challenges from complex inequalities intersecting with each other, including gender inequality, and the impact of climate change and environmental degradation on all, but especially on women and on vulnerable groups (2016, p. 63). These challenges require a multi-pronged policy response. Koehler is interested in how countries move from 'aspired outcomes to implementation of the policies' (p. 63) needed to achieve gender equity and climate justice. Koehler proposes a holistic approach to policy development as a solution. Given their correlation with the SDGs and other policy frameworks, Koehler (p. 64) takes the knowledge domains of income, health and education and the domains of power (inclusive of political and economic), time (time spent in paid and unpaid work, social activities and the 'balance' between) and safety and security (freedom from violence) from the European Gender Equity Index. They build in two additional domains – the care economy, 'to reflect its central role in women's lives, its value to humanity, and importance to "development", and the need to valorise it and make it visible', and the state of the Earth, given that gender equity is preconditioned on a healthy planet (p. 64). Koehler argues that enmeshing these domains together and correlating different policy areas to the new 'policy universe' (p. 64) can eventually change the current logic that underpins policy development and see public policy transform into 'gendered eco-social policy' (p. 65).

Let's finish

This chapter has drawn out the intersections between gender equality and the transformation of how work is organised in contemporary Australia and public and planetary health. Creating a fair and just society is predicated on a healthy planet – our social systems must adapt to a changing physical as well as social environment. Without political intervention, existing social and health inequalities will continue to deepen, and there will be further erosion to the foundational work undertaken towards social justice. The development of policies that have been deliberately designed with reference to their impacts on families and effects for gender equity to target the drivers of inequality are crucial to the interconnected SDGs of achieving gender equality and promoting decent work.

Summary

In this chapter, you have learnt about the health impacts of politics and policy on the family and work. The key areas of focus have included impacts on children and young people, women and the broader family unit, as well as safety at work, equal opportunity, and unpaid care work. The learning objectives for this chapter are summarised here:

- Understand how politics affects the health of families, the effects of politics on work cultures, and the role of state and government in these processes. The chapter provided several examples of how politics affects the health of children and young people, women and families, and work cultures. In addition, the role of the state and government in these processes was discussed. It also argued that governments are responsible for actively fostering inclusive workplaces and supporting the restructuring of care work through well-designed policy instruments.
- Analyse the interconnections between gender equality, the creation of inclusive, sustainable work futures and public health. The chapter discussed the interconnections between gender equality, inclusive, sustainable work futures and public health. The case examples used to illustrate these interconnections included the public health issues of GBV and sexual harassment, the role of paid parental leave policies in creating equal opportunity, and how unpaid carers are supported to provide care to older family members through legislation.
- Assess how effectively policies target the drivers of social and economic inequalities to protect and promote the health and wellbeing of families and women. The chapter debated the effectiveness of current policies in tackling the drivers of social and economic inequalities and protecting and promoting the health and wellbeing of families and women. In doing so, the underlying structures of power driving social phenomena like GBV, sexual harassment and, ultimately, climate change were discussed in reference to the design of policy and the degree of care taken to project the impacts of policy on families and contributions to gender equity.
- Critique the success of contemporary policy initiatives in fostering systemic recognition of and assigning value to unpaid care work by promoting the equitable distribution of this work. This chapter critiqued the success of contemporary policy initiatives in fostering recognition of and assigning value to unpaid care work by promoting the equitable distribution of this work through several case examples. These included paid parental leave, how informal care providers are supported to remain in the paid workforce with the rising need for care within families and communities, and how current policy initiatives fail to encourage a re-distribution of care work between families and the state and between genders.

Tutorial exercises

1   Working in a small team, discuss the key elements that are important to consider regarding paid parental leave schemes (e.g., length of leave, type of wage, eligibility requirements, gender split of entitlement) and why these elements matter in the context of the SDGs. Select a handful of OECD countries. Assign one country to each team member and allow time to review the policy of the assigned country against the elements discussed. Come together and create a comparison chart of the paid parental leave schemes you have reviewed, and, using that chart, see if you can rank these schemes in terms of how well they can progress the SDGs.

2   The tutorial group will be divided into two groups. Each group will take a side in a debate on the topic 'given that the futures of children and young people are the most affected by climate change, 16- and 17-year-olds should have the option to vote in elections at all levels of government'. Teams will have time to discuss and formulate the arguments for their side and potential rebuttal points.

3   Working in a small group, conduct a quick search via the feeds on your social media of recent and trending portrayals of GBV (you may choose to focus on a specific form of GBV). Review these portrayals with each other and notice whose stories may be missing, as well as whose stories are profiled and compare how the stories may be (re)presented in different ways, and to what effect/s.

Further reading

Australian Women Against Violence Alliance. (2021). Criminalisation of coercive control. Issues Paper. Available at: https://awava.org.au/wp-content/uploads/2021/01/FINAL_-2021_-AWAVA-Issues-Paper-Criminalisation-of-Coercive-Control.pdf

Friel, S., Baum, F., Goldfeld, S., Townsend, B., Büsst, C., & Keane, L. (2021). How Australia improved health equity through action on the social determinants of health. In D. Jeyapalan & L. Keane (eds), *Australia in 2030: what is our path to health for all?* (vol. 214). https://doi.org/10.5694/mja2.51020

Hearn, J., Strid, S., Humbert, A.L., & Balkmar, D. (2022). Violence regimes: A useful concept for social politics, social analysis, and social theory. *Theory & Society*, 51(4), 565–594. https://doi.org/10.1007/s11186-022-09474-4

Lowitja Institute. (2022). Indigenous nation building and the political determinants of health and wellbeing. Discussion paper. doi:10.48455/9ace-aw24

Koehler, G. (2016). Tapping the Sustainable Development Goals for progressive gender equity and equality policy? *Gender and Development*, 24(1), 53–68. https://doi.org/10.1080/13552074.2016.1142217

Sustainable Development Solutions Network. (2015). Indicators and a monitoring framework for the Sustainable Development Goals: Launching a data revolution for the Sustainable Development Goals. Report to the Secretary-General of the United Nations. Available at: https://irp-cdn.multiscreensite.com/be6d1d56/files/uploaded/150612-FINAL-SDSN-Indicator-Report1.pdf

United Nations Children's Fund. (2021). Making climate and environment policies for & with children and young people. Climate & Environment discussion paper. Available at: https://www.unicef.org/media/109701/file/Making-Climate-Policies-for-and-with-Children-and-Young-People.pdf

References

Australian Women Against Violence Alliance. (2021). Criminalisation of coercive control. Issues Paper. Available at: https://awava.org.au/wp-content/uploads/2021/01/FINAL_-2021_-AWAVA-Issues-Paper-Criminalisation-of-Coercive-Control.pdf

Bogenschneider, K. (2014). Making a global case for family policy: How families support society and how policies support families. In A. Abela & J. Walker (eds), *Contemporary issues in family studies: Global perspectives on partnerships, parenting and support in a changing world*. Hoboken, NJ: John Wiley & Sons, pp. 369–381.

Brimblecombe, N., Fernandez, J-L., Knapp, M., Rehill, A., & Wittenberg, R. (2018). Review of the international evidence on support for unpaid carers. *Journal of Long-Term Care*, pp. 25–40. https://doi.org/10.31389/jltc.3.

Brimblecombe, N., Pickard, L., King, D., & Knapp, M. (2018). Barriers to receipt of social care services for working carers and the people they care for in times of austerity. *Journal of Social Policy*, 47(2), 215–233. https://doi.org/10.1017/S0047279417000277.

Buckmaster, L. (2022). Comparing the paid parental leave schemes: Social policy. Canberra: Parliament of Australia. Commonwealth of Australia. Available at: https://www.aph.gov.au/About_Parliament/Parliamentary_Departments/Parliamentary_Library/pubs/BriefingBook44p/PaidParentalLeave

Cull, I., Hancock, R. L. A., McKeown, S., Pidgeon, M., & Vedan, A. (2018). Pulling together: A guide for front-line staff, student services, and advisors. Victoria, BC: BCcampus. Available at: https://opentextbc.ca/indigenizationfrontlineworkers/

Cylus, J., Figueras, J., & Normand, C. E. M. (2019). *Will population ageing spell the end of the welfare state?: A review of evidence and policy options*. Geneva: World Health Organization, Regional Office for Europe.

Ferrant, G., Pesando, L. M., & Nowacka, K. (2014). *Unpaid care work: The missing link in the analysis of gender gaps in labour outcomes*. Paris: OECD Development Centre.

Goncharenko, G. (2022). The #MeToo legacy and "the Collective Us": Conceptualising accountability for sexual misconduct at work. *Accounting & Auditing Journal*. https://doi.org/10.1108/AAAJ-01-2022-5642.

Hayes, A., & Higgins, D. (2014). Weaving a common narrative: An introduction to essays on families, policy and the law in Australia. In A. Hayes & D. Higgins (eds), *Families, policy and the law: Selected essays on contemporary issues for Australia*. Melbourne: Australian Institute of Family Studies.

Hayward, B. (2021). *Children, citizenship and environment: #schoolstrike edition* (2nd edn.). New York: Routledge.

Hearn, J., Strid, S., Humbert, A. L., & Balkmar, D. (2022). Violence regimes: A useful concept for social politics, social analysis, and social theory. *Theory & Society*, 51(4), 565–594. https://doi.org/10.1007/s11186-022-09474-4

Hickman, C., Marks, E., Pihkala, P., Clayton, S., Lewandowski, R. E., Mayall, E. E., Wray, B., Mellor, C., & van Susteren, L. (2021). Climate anxiety in children and young people and their beliefs about government responses to climate change: A global survey. *The Lancet Planetary Health*, 5(12), e863–e873. https://doi.org/10.1016/S2542-5196(21)00278–00273.

Humphrey, K. (n.d.). Climate action – It is up to you. Available at: https://onthewards.org/climate-action-it-is-up-to-you/

Hurley, P., Matthews, H., & Pennicuik, S. (2022). Deserts and oases: How accessible is childcare? Melbourne, Victoria: Mitchell Institute, Victoria University.

Huseth-Zosel, A. L., Larson, M., & Nelson, K. (2021). Health effects of the #MeToo movement by gender: Public health implications of a social movement. *Women's Studies International Forum*, 102523. https://doi.org/10.1016/j.wsif.2021.102523.

International Labour Organization. (2022). Social protection floor. Available at: https://www.ilo.org/secsoc/areas-of-work/policy-development-and-applied-research/social-protection-floor/lang–en/index.htm.

International Union for Conservation of Nature. (2020). Gender-based violence and the environment. Available at: https://www.iucn.org/resources/issues-brief/gender-based-violence-and-environment

Jagsi, R. (2018). Sexual harassment in medicine — #MeToo. *The New England Journal of Medicine*, 378 (3), 209–211. https://doi.org/10.1056/NEJMp1715962.

Koehler, G. (2016). Tapping the Sustainable Development Goals for progressive gender equity and equality policy? *Gender and Development*, 24(1). https://doi.org/10.1080/13552074.2016.114221753–68

Lowitja Institute. (2022). Indigenous nation building and the political determinants of health and well-being. Discussion paper. doi:10.48455/9ace-aw24

Lynn, G. (2018). Paid parental leave: An investigation and analysis of Australian paid parental leave frameworks with reference to selected European OECD countries. Master of Laws by Research.

Malatzky, C. (2013). Don't shut up: Australia's first paid parental leave scheme and beyond. *Australian Feminist Studies*, 28(76), 195–211. https://doi.org/10.1080/08164649.2013.789580.

Margaria, A. (2021). Fathers, childcare and COVID-19. *Feminist Legal Studies*, 29(1), 133–144. https://doi.org/10.1007/s10691-021-09454-6.

McDonald, P. (2020). A great awakening with many dangers: What has the# MeToo movement achieved? QUT Centre for Justice Briefing Papers (August), pp. 1–4. Oakley, A. (1980). *Women confined: Towards a sociology of childbirth*. New York: Schocken Books.

OECD. (2017). A good start for equal parenting: Paid parental leave. In Gender Equality in Employment (ed.), *The pursuit of gender equality: An uphill battle*. Paris: OECD Publishing, pp. 199–206. https://doi.org/https://doi.org/10.1787/9789264281318-19-en.

O'Neil, A., Sojo, V., Fileborn, B., Scovelle, A. J., & Milner, A. (2018). The #MeToo movement: An opportunity in public health? *The Lancet (British edition)*, 391, 2587–2589. https://doi.org/10.1016/S0140-6736(18)30991–30997.

Our Watch. (2018). Changing the picture: A national resource to support the prevention of violence against Aboriginal and Torres Strait Islander women and their children. Available at: https://media-cdn.ourwatch.org.au/wp-content/uploads/sites/2/2020/09/20231759/Changing-the-picture-Part-2-AA.pdf.

Parkinson, G. (2019). Morrison to youth on climate change: Don't worry, be happy. *Renew Economy*. Available at: https://reneweconomy.com.au/morrison-to-youth-on-climate-change-dont-worry-be-happy-60523/

Phillips, J., Muller, D., & Lorimer, C. (2015). Domestic violence issues and policy challenges. Research paper series.

Power, K. (2020). The COVID-19 pandemic has increased the care burden of women and families. *Sustainability: Science, Practice, & Policy*, 16(1), 67–73. https://doi.org/10.1080/15487733.2020.1776561.

Raub, A., & Heymann, J. (2021). Progress in national policies supporting the Sustainable Development Goals: Policies that matter to income and its impact on health. *Annual Review of Public Health*, 42(1), 423–437. https://doi.org/10.1146/annurev-publhealth-040119-094151.

Sassler, S., & Lichter, D. T. (2020). Cohabitation and marriage: Complexity and diversity in union-formation patterns. *Journal of Marriage and Family*, 82(1), 35–61. https://doi.org/10.1111/jomf.12617.

Save the Children. (2021). Born into the climate crisis: Why we must act now to secure children's rights. Available at: www.savethechildren.net/born-climate-crisis

Singh, G., Xue, S., & Poukhovski-Sheremetyev, F. (2022). Climate emergency, young people and mental health: time for justice and health professional action. *BMJ Paediatrics Open*, 6(1), e001375. https://doi.org/10.1136/bmjpo-2021-001375.

State Government of Victoria. (2019). Equal opportunity. Available at: https://www.health.vic.gov.au

State of Victoria. (2021). Aboriginal and Torres Strait Islander cultural safety. Department of Health. Available at: https://www.health.vic.gov.au/health-strategies/aboriginal-and-torres-strait-islander-cultural-safety

Sustainable Development Solutions Network. (2012). Indicators and a monitoring framework: Launching a data revolution for the Sustainable Development Goals. Available at: https://indicators.report/targets/5-4/.

UNICEF. (2022). The impacts of climate change put almost every child at risk. Available at: https://www.unicef.org/stories/impacts-climate-change-put-almost-every-child-risk.

United Nations Department of Economic and Social Affairs. (2019). Population dynamics. Available at: https://population.un.org/wpp/Graphs/DemographicProfiles/1500.

van Daalen, K. R., Kallesøe, S. S., Davey, F., Dada, S., Jung, L., Singh, L., Issa, R., Emilian, C. A., Kuhn, I., Keygnaert, I., & Nilsson, M. (2022). Extreme events and gender-based violence: A mixed-methods systematic review. *The Lancet: Planetary Health*, 6(6), e504–e523. Available at: https://doi.org/10.1016/S2542-5196(22)00088–00082.

Weston, R., & Qu, L. (2014). Trends in family transitions, forms and functioning: Essential issues for policy development and legislation. In A. Hayes & D. Higgins (eds), *Families, policy and the law*. Melbourne, Victoria: Australian Institute of Family Studies.

Wilson, A. (2011). Addressing uncomfortable issues: The role of White health professionals in Aboriginal health. Thesis, Flinders University.

2 Diversity and Community

Allyson Mutch and Lisa Fitzgerald

There's good evidence that if people are disempowered, if they have little control over their lives, if they're socially isolated or unable to participate fully in society, then there are biological effects.

—Sir Michael Marmot

Learning objectives

After studying this chapter, you should be able to:

1 Describe the notions of diversity, identity and community.
2 Explore data describing Australia's diversity and critically analyse the experiences of health and climate change for different population groups.
3 Critically analyse the social patterns of health and illness for people from different communities and identity groups in Australia.
4 Define the notions of health inequity and social exclusion and critically analyse how policy and politics socially exclude different communities and identity groups.
5 Critique the notion of identity politics and the processes used in politics and policies to create divisions between communities.

Snapshot

There is a growing movement of anti-trans voices and actions, across the world. In the US, recent legislation in many states has marginalised and breached the human rights of trans and gender diverse people. The UK Government in December 2022 reversed the Gender Recognition Reform Bill, which had removed barriers to transgender people legally changing their gender. The reversal of legislative rights demonstrates how politics can socially exclude groups and undermine fundamental human and citizenship rights. Such actions directly impact the health of trans and gender diverse people, who already experience high rates of stigma, discrimination and poor mental health and wellbeing (Bretherton et al., 2021). In Australia, despite significant social gains for many in the Queer community over the last 20 years, most recently through legislation affirming same-sex marriage, stigma, discrimination, and social exclusion continues, with the focus narrowing to trans and gender diverse people. On 16 March 2023, the hatred and bigotry experienced by transgender and gender diverse people were demonstrated on the steps of Parliament House in Melbourne, at an anti-trans rally. British Anti-trans activist, Kellie Jay Keen Minshull and her 'let women speak' campaigners were joined by a throng of anti-trans supporters, including a vocal group of around 20 Neo-Nazis. Images of scuffles between groups

DOI: 10.4324/9781003315490-5

and police, tear gas, hatred, and distress were shown across mass and social media. Many spoke out against the rally, but some politicians, political candidates and media commentors were vocal in their anti-trans views driving ongoing negative and stigmatising discourse across the media. Every jurisdiction in Australia has some form of anti-discrimination legislation, but there are no anti-vilification laws to protect members of the Queer community from the hate speech and discrimination we are witnessing. We have made progress, but there is still a long way to go to ensure the social inclusion and wellbeing of all members of our community.

Let's begin!

The political determinants of health impact individuals, population groups and communities in a diverse range of direct and indirect ways. This chapter considers the impact of policies and politics on our diversity, as a society made up of many communities and groups linked by distinct and intersecting identities. We begin by developing understanding of who we are and how we live, we then consider our health, acknowledging the unique health outcomes experienced by different population groups. Consideration of health differences leads us to question why these differences occur and to broadly examine the social determinants of health before we narrow our focus to the political determinants. As you work through this book, you will see the many ways the political determinants impact health through consideration of different policies. Within the context of this chapter, we focus specifically on the notion of social exclusion and consider the direct and indirect ways different communities and groups, most notably the LGBTIQA+ community and people living with disability, are excluded from (and included in) participating in social, cultural, economic and political life and the consequences for health. From an understanding of our diversity we move to a consideration of community. Community is a broad term, used frequently, but often without definitional boundaries. We briefly describe the different ways community can be understood and draw on examples from COVID-19 and migration policy to critically consider the impact of politics and policies on the health and wellbeing of our communities.

The health impacts of politics and policy on our diversity

Population

In 2022, Australia was a population of over 26 million people living in an area roughly the size of the mainland of the USA. We are a *diverse* population made up of many identities linked to age, generations, religion, culture, gender, ethnicity, sexuality, and ability. We are an *ageing* population, our average age is 38, with 16% over the age of 65 in 2020 compared to 8.3% in 1970 (AIHW, 2022). Just over 3% of our population are Aboriginal and Torres Strait Islander peoples, with an average age of 24 and only 5.4% aged over 65 (ABS, 2021). We are generally a *connected* population. Most Australians (70.5%) lived in family households and just over half (53%) of them were couples with dependent children in 2021 (ABS, 2021). Nearly 16% of families with children are single parent households – the majority of them are women (ABS, 2021). We are a *multicultural* population. Nearly one-third of us were born overseas with the majority coming from the UK, New Zealand and Asian countries. One in four people are second-generation Australians with one or more parents born overseas. Mandarin is the second most common language spoken at home (ABS, 2021). We are generally a *wealthy* population: one of the wealthiest countries in the Organisation for Economic Co-operation and Development (OECD) (AIHW, 2022). The average salary in 2022 was around $90,000, but in 2019, 20% of the top income earners received six times more money than the bottom 20% – this increased during COVID-19 (Friel et al., 2021). In 2021, 27% of the population received an income support payment from government (e.g., aged pension, Newstart allowance, disability support pension) (AIHW, 2021). We are generally a *home-owning* population. In 2021, most people (67%) owned or were buying their own homes, 26.2% were in the private rental market (up from 18.4% in 1994) and 2.9% were in public housing (down from 5.5% in 1994) (AIHW, 2021). We are in the midst of a housing crisis: nearly half of all low-income households in urban areas were experiencing rental stress (+30% of income on housing costs) in 2017–2018 (AIHW, 2021) – a figure that is estimated to be substantially higher post-COVID-19. In 2021, over 120,000 people (48 per 10,000) were experiencing some form of homelessness (e.g., on the street, boarding houses, temporary accommodation) – but this is estimated to be an under-representation of the situation as many governments placed people in temporary hotel accommodation during the early phases of the pandemic (ABS, 2021).

As one of the driest continents in the world, we are acutely impacted by the changing climate, but this impact is largely mediated by where and how we live and the resources we have. In 2021, most people (72%) were living in major cities and urban areas along the coastline, with 28.0% living in rural and remote areas (less than 2% in (very) remote areas) (ABS, 2021). Many who live in rural areas are accustomed to the challenges of the Australian landscape. Droughts that go for many years push rural communities to the brink. Periods of drought are often followed by intense rain. In the summer of 2019, following a three-year drought, Australia experienced one of its most severe bushfire seasons on record (33 people and an estimated 1.25 billion animals died, over 3,000 homes were lost). This was soon followed by a significant flood in 2022 that covered much of eastern Australia. These events created an acute and broad awareness of the impact of climate change on our communities, but, as we will see, the impact was not felt equally.

Indigenous perspective: The impact of climate change in Torres Strait

Torres Strait Islander peoples are the traditional owners of 274 islands and live on 16 islands across the north of Australia. The increasing impact of climate change on rising sea levels is threatening homes, sacred cultural sites, hunting sites and the many traditions and cultural practices of communities (Lyons, 2022). Poorer health outcomes are also being experienced in Torres Strait Islander communities linked to increasing storms and cyclones that inundate homes and food crops, more frequent droughts and higher ambient temperatures that cause heat stress, and increasing rates of mosquito borne communicable diseases. In 2019, eight Torres Strait Elders lodged a complaint with the United Nations Human Rights Committee (UNHRC) against the Australian Government for failing to take action on climate change which is damaging their livelihoods, culture and way of life (Lyons, 2022). The UNHRC found the Australian Government's lack of action, inadequate policies and climate denial over many decades had failed to protect the Torres Strait community, violating their human rights and placing them at significant risk. The Committee argued a healthy ecosystem was critical to the community's ability to maintain cultural practices and wellbeing and that the Government must act and ensure the rights of First Nations peoples are upheld in climate policy development and planning (Lyons, 2022).

The diversity of our population is closely linked to the diversity of health experiences and health care needs. The Australian Institute of Health and Welfare's (AIHW) biennial report on

Australia's health provides a detailed summary of our health and illness (AIHW, 2022). Life expectancy is mixed across the population, but in general we have one of the longest life expectancies across OECD countries (AIHW, 2022). A teenage boy (15 years) in 2018–2020 would expect to live to 81.6 years and a teenage girl to 85.7 years (AIHW, 2022), but life expectancy and premature mortality rates are not experienced equally across our population. Men tend to die at an earlier age than women, and if you are a man experiencing higher rates of marginalisation and disadvantage, your rate of premature death is 1.8 times that of men who experience higher levels of advantage. First Nations' life expectancy is lower than the general population but has been increasing – an Indigenous boy born in 2015–2017 has a life expectancy of 71.6 years, and a girl 75.6 years (AIHW, 2022). For people living in rural areas, premature mortality rates and health outcomes are poorer than their urban counterparts: life expectancy rates are up to seven years less (AIHW, 2022). People living with developmental disability can have a life expectancy up to 20 years shorter than the general population. Infant mortality rates have improved over the last hundred years dropping from 65.7 in 1927 to 3.3 deaths per 1,000 live births in 2019, but we were ranked 20 out of 38 OECD countries because infant mortality rates are still unacceptably high among some population groups – in 2015–2017 infant mortality was 6.2 among First Nations babies (AIHW, 2022). The leading causes of death for Australian children were injury (33%) and cancer (19%) (AIHW, 2022). Among adults, coronary heart disease was the leading cause of death for men and dementia was the leading cause for women in 2020. Lung cancer, cerebrovascular disease (e.g., stroke), breast and prostate cancer were also in the top five causes of death in 2020 (AIHW, 2022). The increasing age of our population parallels rising rates of dementia and cognitive decline: over 400,000 people (15 per 1,000; 84 per 1,000 for people over 65) were estimated to be living with dementia in 2022 – two-thirds were women. The rate of dementia is expected to more than double in the next 30 years (AIHW, 2022). Poorer mental health has been experienced by two in five people our population, with anxiety (17.0%) and affective disorders such as depression (8.0%) the most common conditions (AIHW, 2022). Social isolation and loneliness play a critical role in our mental health. During COVID-19 around half the population reported feeling lonely, up from one in three in 2001–2009 (AIHW, 2021). Psychological distress and use of mental health services also increased during the COVID-19 pandemic (AIHW, 2022).

In terms of the standard risk factors that frequently dominant health discourse, we are experiencing increasing rates of weight gain. In 2017–2018 one in three adults were overweight (36%) and nearly one in three were obese (31%): 75.0% of people in rural and remote areas and 76.5% of people in our most socioeconomically marginalised areas were experiencing obesity or were overweight. In 2017, we ranked eighth in the OECD for increasing weight and 17 out of 38 countries for alcohol consumption, but in 2019 we were one of the lowest smoking countries in the OECD – just over 11% of our population smoked (AIHW, 2022).

Let's think!

What role do you think the commercial determinants of health play in increasing rates of weight gain in high-income countries like Australia? We've provided some excellent recommended readings and podcasts led by Professor Sharon Friel. These are listed in the References and are available for you to draw on to consider this question.

Equity and exclusion

As the previous discussion illustrates, we are connected and divided by a broad range of factors that impact our health. Importantly, we can see experiences of health and different rates of illness are unevenly distributed and social patterned with some population groups experiencing poorer health outcomes than others (Bambra et al., 2005). If we were to dig a little deeper, we can see differences in health are connected to different levels of education, unemployment or underemployment, locality, types of occupations, income and many other factors of described as the social determinants of health. For example, when we consider the impact of climate change on health, we can see that many in our society do not have the social and economic resources needed to navigate the changing environment and are more susceptible to health inequities as a result (Friel, 2022). Those who are older, have disabilities, are poor and socially marginalised are most acutely impacted as they are 'the least able to adapt to the changing climate, unable to escape the [floods,] fires and heat, and live in dwellings and environments that amplify its effects' (Friel, 2022, p. 466). But while public health researchers have traditionally focused on the social determinants when considering health inequities, many are now arguing we must also consider the political nature of these determinants and how they impact health (Bambra et al., 2005). In short, what are the political determinants driving the social determinants of health? Health inequities are inherently tied to politics and policy because the structural, social, environmental and commercial conditions for health are amenable to political responses and dependent on, and directly affected by, political (in)action (Bambra et al., 2005). In other words, past, current and future policies are intricately tied to the health inequities experienced by the groups who are socially excluded from participation in our social world.

Let's refresh!

By now you will be familiar with the term, the social determinants of health. Some within public health are increasingly describing the social determinants as social risk factors linked to poorer health outcomes (e.g., measures of health literacy are correlated with poor health outcomes), but such reductionist descriptions oversimplify the complex and intersecting processes driving health inequities. More broadly, we see the social determinants as an umbrella term that incorporates the social, political, economic and commercial processes linked how we are born, work, live and age. They include the intermediate material and psychosocial factors that impact health, such as social support, living and working conditions, and stress which in turn are driven by the broader structural determinants. These structural determinants, embedded in economic and political systems, institutions and ideologies, are the engine room driving economic, social and cultural processes that produce and distribute systems of power and wealth. Through these structural determinants institutionalised forms of racism, sexism, gender-bias, classism, and ageism are constantly (re)produced generating social and health inequities (Bambra et al., 2005). Summarising these processes and relationships, the WHO Commission on the Social Determinants of Health (CSDH 2008: prelude) described the social determinants of health as: 'the circumstances in which people grow, live, work, and age, and the systems put in place to deal with illness. The conditions in which people live and die are, in turn, shaped by political, social, and economic forces.'

If you are not confident with your knowledge of the social determinants of health or would like to deepen your understanding, we would recommend the seminal reference by Solar and Irwin (2010), listed in the Further reading at the end of this chapter.

To expand our knowledge of the impact of the political determinants on the health of key population groups we must establish a clearer understanding of what we mean by the terms inequity and social exclusion. Let's begin by thinking about inequity. What is inequity? Is it the same as inequality? When we talk about equality, or more frequently inequality we are identifying the many ways in which people and groups experience difference. These differences may be related to biological or genetic characteristics, for example as we age we are more likely to experience poorer health and increasing rates of disease as our bodies negotiate wear and tear. Similarly, if we are born with a particular condition or have a genetic predisposition to a particular condition such as Huntington's disease or multiple sclerosis, we will experience poorer health than others in the community. We can also experience inequalities based on where we live, the types of work we do (e.g., manual labour, that is poorly paid and located in a high impact workplace, versus working as a professional in a high-income job), our gender, skin colour or cultural background. These inequalities are frequently associated with experiences of ill health that stem from structural and social contexts that are socially *unjust and unfair*. It is at this point that we turn to the term inequity and can see inequities, those differences that are unjust and unfair, are embedded in policies and political systems that support the privilege of certain groups, maintaining inequities in power in our social systems and socially excluding some from participation in economic, social, cultural and political life.

Understanding *social exclusion* is foundational for our understanding of equity and the political determinants of health providing a lens from which to consider the different ways in which politics and policies exclude different groups and maintain systems of power and inequity. Marmot and Wilkinson (2005) define social exclusion as: 'not only to the economic hardship of relative economic poverty, but also incorporates the notion of the process of marginalization—how individuals come, through their lives, to be excluded and marginalized from various aspects of social and community life'. White (1998) outlines four elements of social exclusion. The first connects to exclusion from *participating in civil society*, which is linked to regulations or legislation that limit access to the rights and duties associated with citizenship. Some groups are substantively disconnected from political participation due to forms of exclusion that emanate from systemic forms of discrimination connected to gender, race, disability, sexuality, ethnicity and/or religion (e.g., in Australia the right to vote was only given to women in 1901 and First Nations people in 1962). The second form of social exclusion relates to a *failure to supply social goods*, more specifically the failure of the state to directly or indirectly supply social goods and services that meet basic needs. For example, access to some forms of healthcare in rural/remote communities (e.g., obstetrics care), or to translation services that support participation in health education for people who do not speak English, lack of emergency housing for people who are homeless, or the inability to access essential medications listed on the Pharmaceutical Benefits Scheme (PBS) for migrants with certain types of visas. The third form of social exclusion relates to limiting participation in *social production*. White describes this form of exclusion as ideological, as it excludes people and groups from discourses of power restricting participating in the production of cultural and social activities, norms and processes. For example, particular groups may be labelled as unacceptable (e.g., asylum seekers who arrive by boat), in need of management and control (e.g., people receiving unemployment benefits who must adhere to stringent job searching protocols, income management and cashless debit cards made compulsory in some First Nations and marginalised communities). The final form of exclusion describes *exclusion from social consumption* which excludes people from economic participation, creating financial hardship and limiting income generation. Linked to industrial regulations and deregulation of labour markets – exclusion from the labour market not only impacts livelihoods, but also social identity (e.g., an 'able-bodied' citizen is one who economically contributes to society). Exclusion from social consumption has implications for health, not only through access to economic resources, but also through the unequal distribution of access to labour markets (e.g., workplaces that offer poor reward, limited levels of control and precarious, unstable or insecure employment). It is critical to note that these forms of exclusion do not occur in isolation but are frequently intersecting and mutually reinforcing. Importantly, as the snapshot we presented at the beginning of the chapter illustrated, social exclusion is not fixed, but evolves and changes in line with changing social, cultural and political contexts, differentially targeting some groups in explicit and implicit ways at different times.

Identity

Let's do

Think about the notion of identity and write down all the different ways you might identify yourself? If you're reading this textbook, you might be a student? You will live in a particular location and connect to a certain place (e.g., rural community, regional area, urban area). You may identify based on age and feel a sense of connection to a particular generation? You may identify with a particular gender or identify as non-binary? A particular sexuality? Ethnicity or culture? There are many ways we can identify, rarely is it based on a singular characteristic, although at different time points or in different contexts one aspect of your identity might stand out more than at other times. There are no limitations, your list can be as short or as long as you think.

Now you are equipped with some tools to help you critically consider the impacts of policy and politics on different groups, let's develop a clearer understanding of the notion of identity and consider some groups who are frequently excluded because of their identity. Identity is often seen as something so natural, innate, but social identities, that is, the ways groups internalise established social categories, are forged in the social sphere and temporal relations of past, present, and future understandings of identities. Identity is spoken through a range of categories and positions (e.g., gender, sexuality, generational, faith, culture, social class). Identity is relational, formed and played out in relation to those who are like us, and those who are different. Identity is context-specific to time and place – to be a Queer young person in Australia in 2023 is very different to being a gay young man in the 1970s, when homosexuality was criminalised and medicalised, as we examine in the spotlight on the 1978 Gay and Lesbian march in Sydney.

Spotlight: Advocacy action

1978: The first Gay and Lesbian march (Mardi Gras) in Sydney

Mark Gillespie provides an account of his experiences of the 1978 protest march (the predecessor to today's Mardi Gras) to advocate recognition and awareness of the rights of LGBTIQA+ people. His account highlights the many ways members of the Queer community, and their Allies were social excluded and discriminated against by government institutions and policies. The march was organised to bring people together to generate collective action, and call for legislative change reversing laws that prohibited homosexuality and policed people's private lives. During the protest, 54 people were arrested – all lost their jobs and some lost housing after their names and addresses were published in the paper – national sex-discrimination laws that would have prohibited such discrimination were not passed until 1984.

On a cold Saturday night in Sydney on June 24, 1978, a number of gay men, lesbians and transgender people marched into the pages of Australian social history. I was one of them. Several protests and demonstrations were organised during June that year to commemorate the 1969 Stonewall riot in New York and to demand civil rights for Australian lesbians and gay men … At Taylor Square, where we assembled, I was impressed by the turnout (a report in The Australian estimated the crowd at about 1,000 people at this early stage of the night). The early rainbow nature of the movement was evident, with transgender and Aboriginal people and people from migrant backgrounds all mixing in. We were a diverse and spirited group of a few hundred mostly younger men and women ready to march down Oxford Street to Hyde Park, along a strip that was becoming the centre of gay life in the city. The atmosphere was more one of celebration than protest. Little did we know then that, by the end of the night, many of us would be traumatised and our lives changed forever. As a young émigré in my twenties, from the Queensland bush, like many gay men and lesbians from the country in those days, I was, in effect, an internally displaced person. We were refugees in our own country. All through history, cities have offered people like me a measure of escape from oppression and persecution. Having arrived in Sydney seeking refuge from the never-ending police state of mind that was life under the Joh Bjelke-Petersen Queensland government, I was renting a studio flat in Crown Street, Darlinghurst, at the time. Living a 'double life' was a means of survival. Gay people's lives were wrapped in stigma and shame. The real unspoken tragedy of the times was the loss of the lives of so many wonderful young people who struggled with their sexual identities and, unable to deal with all the pain and shame inflicted on them, ended up committing suicide … The discriminatory attitude of the police and the violence they meted out to us seemed to represent in highly symbolic and condensed form the very pain, humiliation and suffering that society as a whole constantly inflicted on us as lesbians and gay men.

Acknowledging the role of multiple identities in the formation of ourselves we must look to the notion of *intersectionality* to understand connections between identities. We are all characterised by multiple and intersecting identities. Kimberlé Crenshaw, a lawyer and academic, was one of the first people to coin the term 'intersectionality'. She argued experiences of gender are not universal but embedded in a person's multiple and interconnect identities. Crenshaw also argued experiences of identity are not just created and experienced by individuals, but also stem from social systems and structures – the ways norms and values are produced and reproduced. Through multiple identities we experience multiple forms of social exclusion which impact how people navigate social, economic, and political systems, but not all identities are marginalising, some are sites of advantage and power.

Hall describes identity as the *meeting place* between subjective processes inscribed in the ways we live our identities and the social systems and structures that position us (Hall & Du Gay, 1996). We forge our identities within powerful social systems and institutions (e.g., education, politics, religion), that inscribe what are 'acceptable' identities and what identities are marginalised and stigmatised. Politics is an important institution of power in inscribing such discourses. For example, Australian legal and political institutions based on colonial systems have had ongoing ramifications for First Nations peoples' sovereignty and self-determination.

Actors within the political system are in powerful positions to provide meaning, representation and control, and to 'other' identity groups. People who identify with the LGBTIQA+ community provide a stark example of the impact of 'othering' on health with substantial evidence documenting health inequities, including high rates of physical and mental morbidity and premature mortality (Badgett, 2011). Poorer health outcomes experienced by the Queer community are linked to a range of social and political determinants that embed discrimination and stigma to people's everyday lives. Historically, members of the LGBTIQ+ community in Australia and globally, have been social excluded from participating in civil society and social production (White, 1998; Badgett, 2011). For over 400 years, LGBTIQA+ people have experienced social, medical and legal oppression, vilification, stigma and discrimination. Change has only really begun to take place in the last 50 years in Australia (in 2023, homosexuality was still outlawed in over 60 countries) starting with the decriminalisation of homosexual acts in South Australia in 1975 and concluding with legislative change in Tasmania in 1997 (following legal challenges including representation to the UN). These examples from the Queer community serve to represent how social identities are excluded, but they also demonstrate how groups can challenge the established social order (see the description of the policy processes linked to the HIV pandemic), although any contestation of identities involves the negotiation of power relations, as Okoli argues:

> Social identities are relational; groups typically define themselves in relation to other. This is because identity has little meaning without the 'other'. So, by defining itself as a group defines others. Identity is rarely claimed or assigned for its own sake. These definitions of self and others have purpose and consequences. They are tied to rewards and punishment, which may be material or symbolic. There is usually an expectation of gain or loss as a consequence of identity claims. This is why identities are contested. Power is implicated here, and because groups do not have equal powers to define both self and other, the consequences reflect these power differentials.
>
> (2003, p. 2)

Spotlight: Policy process

Australia's response to HIV

Policy and politics can be used to effectively and positively impact the health of some groups. HIV in Australia is an important example of this. Since the start of the epidemic in the 1980s, Australia has been internationally recognised as a policy leader in its response to HIV/AIDS. From the beginning of the identification of HIV/AIDs in 1982, federal and state governments responded proactively and HIV in Australia became a critical success story in prevention, partnerships and community action. National HIV strategies (the first developed in 1989), were grounded in a strong partnership approach that involved bipartisan political support (i.e., agreement between the then Labor Government and opposition Liberal/National coalition) and collaboration between communities affected by HIV. The partnerships model drew on the Ottawa Charter and supported a social public health approach advocating for harm minimisation (e.g., needle and syringe exchange programmes), mobilization of affected communities (e.g., gay men, people who inject drugs and sex workers), public and peer health promotion and sex education, and research and surveillance to ensure a strong evidence base. Over the 40 years of the epidemic, we have effectively drawn on these collaborations to respond to the changing profile of HIV to achieve some of the lowest HIV infection rates across the developed world. The

HIV pandemic galvanised the LGBTIQ+ community re-channelling the social movement of the 1970s into a consumer movement to improve health care, working actively with politics and policy to reduce the impact of the pandemic in Australia. Unfortunately, many governments around the world did not follow this approach resulting in much higher prevalence rates and significant inequities in health outcomes.

Finally, we turn to the notion of identity politics – organised groups excluded because of something important to their sense of self, such as race, gender, sexuality, and cultural identity. The Indigenous Rights movement, the Feminist movement, (including the #MeToo movement), the LGBTIQA+ movement and the disability movement, are examples of identity politics in Australia. The community response to HIV we outlined is an excellent example of identity politics, where the Queer community worked in partnership with government to develop policy responses to HIV grounded in the rights of LGBTQI+. Actors within the political system can attack identity politics. Pauline Hanson, of the Australia First political party, is an example of a politician who condemns certain groups defining their own versions of identity (such as First Nations, Muslim, migrant and refugee people). For Hanson, diversity of identities is 'other' to 'Australian values'. John Howard's Coalition Government consistently othered asylum seekers, a discourse that has continued across our society for over 20 years. Political discourses and policies which other identity groups, impact broader social understanding of those groups, as well as people's own sense of identity and belonging which impacts health and wellbeing, as First Nations Filipino singer/song-writer Mojo Ju Ju described in a radio interview:

> As a young child, I remember being in the playground being taunted, and I think anyone out there that grew up Asian in Australia during the 80's and 90's knows that Asians were often public enemy number one. I went through puberty when Pauline Hanson became a household name, and I came of age under the government of John Howard. It wasn't a time that was particularly favourable for any kind of migrant family. And I don't think it's changed all that much, the focus has just changed to different identities.
>
> (Carmona, 2018)

Global context: Marriage equality

The negative health effects of social exclusion and discrimination on members of the Queer community have previously been described; however, in this consideration of the global context of marriage equality, we focus on the circumstances and processes leading to legal recognition of same-sex marriage, and consider the impact political debate, identity politics and legislative processes can have on health. Legal recognition of same-sex relationships is critical in the path towards social inclusion and civic participation for members of the LGBTIQA+ community. By allowing members of the community to participate in marriage, a central social institution in western democracies, governments are providing access to the same economic and legal rights as heterosexual couples (Badgett, 2011). By February 2023, 34 countries had legalised same-sex marriage (Drabble et al., 2021), but it wasn't only in April 2001 that the Netherlands became the first country to enact same-sex marriage laws. Belgium and key states in Canada followed in 2003 and the US in 2015 following a Supreme Court ruling (Badgett, 2011). Most countries had brought about legislative change through parliamentary processes, but in Ireland the decision was made via popular vote in 2015 following a national referendum – a significant step for a staunchly Catholic country. Australia has been slower to move. Between 2004 and 2017, there were 22 unsuccessful bills submitted through Australia's parliament to change the Marriage Act to recognise LGBTIQ relationships. The Howard Government staunchly rejected same-sex relationships introducing a bill in 2004 that defined marriage as a union between a man and a woman and refusing to recognise marriages and unions conducted overseas. In 2017, a survey was proposed by the Turnbull Coalition Government to bypass ongoing opposition. The non-compulsory marriage equality postal survey was supported by 61.6% of the country (79.5% of the population voted) and was quickly legislated through the introduction of a private members bill (some members of the government abstained from voting). The public debate that preceded the vote was extremely damaging for the Queer community (there are parallels with the Voice to Parliament). Research reported experiences of stress, anger, sadness, a sense of dehumanising, disconnection, fear of personal safety and a heightened awareness of social stigma. Two years on, there was some shift in the experiences of surveyed participants with many reporting broader community resources and support, greater confidence and acceptance by family and friends, and a stronger sense of connection across the Queer community (Casey et al., 2022).

Disability

Our discussion so far has highlighted the unfair and unjust ways different groups are impacted by politics and policy, but this examination would not be complete without consideration of a key group of people which continues to experience poorer health outcomes and high levels of exclusion. People living with disability are one of the most socially marginalised groups in our community. Disability is defined in many ways encompassing diverse abilities. The ABS defines disability according to measurement and prevalence: 'Disability refers to any person with a limitation, restriction, or impairment, which has lasted, or is likely to last, for at least six months and restricts everyday activities' (ABS, 2013, cited in Habibis, 2019). Critics argue such definitions are inadequate and fail to recognise the social nature of disability. As Habibis argues:

> [Disability is] a socially constructed and contested term (for which the definition has varied over time and between cultures) that broadly refers to physical and/or mental limitations, restrictions or impairments that can be chronic or last for a sustained period of time.
>
> (2019, p. 327)

Importantly, Habibis draws attention to the social model of disability which distinguishes impairment and disability. The former relates to the physical condition, whereas disability is the social construction of impairment. Drawing on this distinction, the social model of disability is embedded in a human rights framework and argues impairment does not justify differential treatment, but instead advocates that environments and policies must ensure people living with impairment are not socially excluded from processes of social production and consumption.

Over four million people in Australia live with a disability, experiencing some of the worst health outcomes in our community (AIHW, 2022). For some, the impact of living with impairment is profound, requiring ongoing care and support, for others care is maintained by self-management with some/limited support. Historically, government policies in the areas of profound physical, intellectual and behavioural disability were based on extreme forms of social exclusion. In the 1970s, institutionalisation and segregation from all forms of social and civic participation were the norm, with a number of parliamentary inquiries documenting harrowing accounts of abuse and violation of basic human rights (Habibis, 2019). Government policies of deinstituionalisation followed, but the stark under-resourcing of community providers and continued reliance on informal care demonstrates ongoing processes of social exclusion, not only in relation to the failure to supply social goods but also through the development of inadequate policy arrangements that address social exclusion (Habibis, 2019).

Despite these significant limitations, the Federal Government has attempted to improve the lives of people living with disability through the development of the National Disability Insurance Scheme (NDIS). The NDIS was recommended following a Productivity Commission inquiry into disability care in 2010–2011 that identified significant underfunding, inefficiencies, fragmentation and little opportunity for community participation. The Commission argued the NDIS should reduce the (financial) barriers that prevent people with disability and their carers/families from participating in the social, economic and cultural life; raising awareness of the issues that impact people with disabilities and providing comprehensive, individually tailored services, supports and information. Critical to the implementation of the Scheme was an advocacy campaign run by a grass-roots organisation – Every Australian Counts, which documented the lives and experiences of people living with disability (see Further reading). The NDIS was passed through parliament in 2012 (Habibis, 2019). It provides broad based, tailored support to over 550,000 people. Yet, despite clear benefits the Scheme relies on a market model to address the needs of individuals rather than a social model that challenges structural inequalities and forms of exclusion and discrimination. The care people receive is dependent on market providers, but current investigations into corruption, over charging and inequities in access associated with complex application and management processes clearly demonstrate the limitations of the scheme as a policy response to the needs of people living with disability.

Limelight: Advocacy for people living with disability

The United Nations Convention of the Rights of Persons with Disabilities (CRPD) is an example of advocacy at the broadest systems level. Ratified by 126 countries, including Australia in 2008, the CRPD enshrines rights to education, social participation, work and employment, and adequate standard of living and social protection. But these rights must be enacted to ensure meaningful improvements in people's health and wellbeing. Stigma can lead to discrimination and the undermining of rights. Advocacy is an essential part of addressing and reducing stigma. Advocacy can take place at the individual or systems level. Individual advocacy broadly refers to 'standing up for' a person to represent and protect their interests and rights whereas systems level advocacy refers to wider legislation, policy and practice to improve the rights and wellbeing of excluded groups. Thinking about adults living with disability it's critical that you are aware of these ways in which this population group are socially excluded and experience higher rates of poor health, social disadvantage and social stigma. As a future public health practitioner, you will engage in advocacy at individual and systems levels and must consider how your role can contribute to improving the wellbeing of people living with disability. Think critically, what actions can you take to advocate for the health and wellbeing of all?

The health impacts of politics and policy on our community

Types

> Community is an important concept for social change because it helps us to see that social change requires a change in some of the most important stories, we tell ourselves. Social change requires that we rewrite our communal narratives. Social change is change in community.
>
> (Lowe, 2021)

Communities are impacted by politics and policies, which subsequently influence health and wellbeing. *Community* is a term we know – we are all part of communities; however, it is often poorly defined. Contemporary understandings highlight the complex and varied nature of communities. Communities can be understood as a social unit with commonality of place, norms, values, or identity, a feeling and/or set of relationships among people. People form and maintain communities to meet common needs. Members of community have trust and care for each other, share experiences, values, belonging, identity, and history. Community has a relational understanding, it implies similarity and difference, as we define our communities in relation to others (Chavis & Lee, 2015). We are all part of multiple communities – based on where we live, our nationality, politics, ethnicity, faith, age, gender, hobbies, sexual identity. We can sometimes experience tensions between communities of belonging when communities, defined by their identities, clash (e.g., LGBTIQ+ and faith-based communities). Chavis and Lee (2015) describe communities as Russian Matryoshka dolls: communities sit within communities. Within our local communities are many diverse communities of interest (e.g., based on age, gender, interests, faith). Our local communities link into broader communities (state, national and international and virtual communities). Communities can include formal institutions (such as schools, government) and informal institutions (helpers and leaders, service clubs). Communities are where politics and policies get 'under the skin', where we experience the impact of policies on our everyday lives (e.g., poor environmental regulation, climate stressors and health in the Torres Strait Islands as we discussed earlier).

Let's think

Why is community important when thinking about the political determinants of health? How do politics and policies use community to achieve certain outcome and agendas? Think about a public health policy you are most familiar with – how is the notion of community defined and used within the context of that policy? Are there distinct identity groups that have been identified?

The term 'community' is used and misused in politics – drawn on in policy conversations to drive policy change (e.g., the discourse that the proposed 2024 Federal tax cuts which will mainly benefit the top 20% income earners will benefit 'the community'). The term community can be used in policy and politics to define, stigmatise, and marginalise some communities, or groups within communities, causing social exclusion. For example, historically, unemployment policy in Australia has understood unemployment as a moral failing of the individual to be punished rather than supported, stigmatising and socially excluding unemployed people from social consumption, and full participation in society (Klein, 2020). However, it is important to note that it is within communities where social change to advance equity and social inclusion occurs and where your role as a public health advocate will come to the fore. Lowe (2021) stresses that social change *is* community (e.g., same-sex marriage legislation to improve the rights of people from the LGBTIQA+ community). It is within community where abstract notions of human rights and equity are brought to life through practices of people, and the politics of narrative construction about who gets to belong, whose voice counts, who gets to tell their own story. The following discussion of COVID-19 and migration policy provides a critical example of the best and worst ways in which politics engages with community, bringing us together but also excluding, discriminating and sometimes dividing us.

COVID-19

> It was the best of times, it was the worst of times, it was the age of wisdom, it was the age of foolishness, it was the epoch of belief, it was the epoch of incredulity, it was the season of light, it was the season of darkness, it was the spring of hope, it was the winter of despair
> (Charles Dickens, 1859, *A Tale of Two Cities*)

Dickens' famous quote could not be more appropriate for a discussion of COVID-19. The pandemic was a critical time that is continuing to impact Australian and global communities. COVID-19 was a magnifying glass on social and health inequities, but it also showed how quickly policy makers and politicians can act, when needed. On 27 February 2020, then Prime Minister Scott Morrison spoke on national television to announce the activation of the Health Sector Emergency Response Plan for Novel Coronavirus. On 11 March 2020, the WHO declared COVID-19 a global pandemic. The Government's early response was quick and decisive – a National Cabinet of the prime minister, premiers and health ministers from all states and territories was formed and quickly implemented quarantines and mandatory lockdowns, restricting movement across borders, business operations and personal movements. The Federal Government acknowledged the significant impact the virus would have on the Australian community, but using a discourse of unity Morrison and others claimed: 'we are all in this together' and needed to protect every member of our community from the deaths and disease we were witnessing across the globe. The national policy response was broad, comprehensive, and for some, generous. Multiple economic support programs providing temporary economic and welfare payments for businesses and individuals were implemented in anticipation of the significant personal and social costs of the shutdowns (Friel et al., 2021). Health system, adjustments included suspension of many non-urgent health services and surgeries, but telehealth and e-script services were substantially expanded and funded through Medicare. These were unprecedented times that significantly disrupted social, economic and health landscapes and provided significant impetus for government action and response.

Limelight

As part of the COVID-19 pandemic response, the Newstart unemployment allowance, which had been frozen for 25 years under the Howard Coalition Government, socially excluding many from social and economic consumption and participation was increased by $550 a fortnight substantially lifting many out of poverty in the short term (Friel et al., 2021). Consider arguments for keeping the Newstart unemployment allowance at this increased rate. What benefit might this have for those on Newstart and for the broader community?

As the pandemic continued, early discourse that 'COVID-19 does not discriminate' was quickly rebuked as the impact of the pandemic was differentially experienced by the most marginalised in the community (e.g., early deaths among elderly people in residential facilities highlighted the structural and policy failures of the aged care system and the ways government policy has excluded older people by failing to supply the social goods needed for their day-to-day care). The inherent divisiveness and inequities of access embedded in many of the government's COVID-19 emergency policies were also revealed as key population groups across the community were excluded from accessing critical payments (e.g., temporary visa holders and international students stranded due to border closures were ineligible for welfare payments despite losing employment) (Friel et al., 2021). As the pandemic continued into its second year, many social, political and economic challenges were magnified. Globally and in Australia, COVID-19 had served to re-centre the role of clinicians, public health practitioners and researchers following a period of ongoing critique and de-legitimation (e.g., the Trump administration initially claimed that COVID-19 was a 'hoax' and reduced funding for the Center for Disease Control, which, many argued, undermined their pandemic preparedness). But as we moved towards the end of 2020 and into 2021, political agendas and ideologies began again to sideline scientists and public health researchers creating divisions across the community. As the vaccine roll-out began we saw increasing debates and division about safety (particularly due to early concerns linking the AstraZeneca vaccine to blood clots) and the mandatory nature of vaccination, which led sections of the community, including some vocal politicians to question the evidence and express concerns about their civil rights. These divisions in the community were in many ways reinforced by political ruptures, as the Federal Coalition Government was critical of the actions of some of the state (Labor) governments, particularly Victoria, Queensland and Western Australia that maintained border closures and implemented lockdowns and movement restrictions when the national government was trying to open the country.

Spotlight: Other determinants

As the vaccine roll-out continued, many of the most marginalised in the community, who were the most susceptible to COVID-19 complications, including First Nations people, people with disabilities and older people, were left unprotected, with significant consequences, as our account of First Nations communities in rural NSW demonstrates. How do you think the vaccine roll-out could have been improved? In particular, think about public messaging and issues of access, such as cost and availability. What other determinants of health are evident here?

Overall, our national response to COVID-19, which had started with a discourse of unity and community connectedness, moved to a discourse of distrust and division as political leaders, health practitioners and researchers and broader ideological groups in the community became submerged in critiques of the vaccine roll-out, health systems failures and mandatory vaccination policies that undermined civil liberties. The mortality rate grew steadily during this time, linked most clearly to mutations in the virus and health systems pressures, but one must also critically reflect on the divisive discourse and adequacy of the broader political response.

Indigenous perspective: The experience of COVID-19

Australia's response to COVID-19 demonstrated the best and worst of policy action in First Nations communities. Early on, Indigenous leaders, researchers and healthcare professionals recognised that fundamental shortfalls in resources, along with the structural determinants that meant the impact of COVID-19 on First Nations communities would be potentially catastrophic (Crooks et al., 2020). Government and Indigenous leaders came together to establish the Aboriginal and Torres Strait Islander Advisory Group on COVID-19, which was co-chaired by the National Aboriginal Community Controlled Health Organisation and included a broad and locally responsive membership. The Advisory Group worked in partnership to lead a culturally embedded, equity driven and strengths-based response to minimise the impact of COVID-19 on First Nations communities. This early response demonstrated the effectiveness of First Nations leadership and partnerships (Crooks et al., 2020). However, as the vaccine roll-out began, shortage of resources in community and the government's substantial lack of investment in health and social care services highlighted significant challenges. Indigenous leaders and medical services had argued that First Nations peoples needed to be identified as a priority group for vaccination, but the lack of health systems, structures and workforce hampered the roll out (Williamson, 2021). As the pandemic moved into its second and third wave, issues of poor housing and overcrowding also amplified the spread and impact of the virus (Williamson, 2021). Communities in western NSW were particularly impacted. Public health responses only served to deepen historical experiences of mistrust, institutional racism and fundamental issues of social exclusion through the government's failure to provide basic social goods (Williamson, 2021).

Migration

Over the last 100 years millions of people have been displaced from their homelands by war –the upheaval and destruction caused by the First and Second World Wars, followed by the Vietnam and Korean Wars have seen the significant displacement of many people. More recently, we are facing a substantial increase in the number of people seeking asylum as a consequence of war and conflict in Syria, Afghanistan, and Iraq along with civil conflicts in Columbia and Sudan. In 2012, just over 40 million people were displaced, by 2022 100 million people had been forced to flee their homes and homelands (UNHCR, 2023). Concerningly, the UNHCR identifies displacement caused by climate changes as one of the most pressing issues of our time estimating that climate refugees will quadrupole over the next 10 years (UNHCR 2023). Columbia, Turkey, Pakistan and Uganda are some of the countries most engaged in providing a safe haven to asylum seekers, whereas Australia's response is one of the weakest.

Let's refresh

What is the difference between someone who is a refugee and someone seeking asylum?

Australia has a long-standing history of exclusion of refugees and people seeking asylum. One of the earliest acts of the new Federal parliament following federation in 1901 was the establishment of the Immigration Restriction Act. This Act, also known as the White

Australia Policy, substantially excluded access to 'non-white' migrants (only 0.25% of Australian residents at the time were non-white), but it wasn't until the 1950s that things began to change. Our need to 'populate or perish' during the nation-building period that followed the Second World War saw a shift in policy to allow an increase in the number of southern Europeans from Italy, Greece and Crete – government efforts to secure sufficient numbers from the UK had been unsuccessful. In 1973, the white Australia policy was finally dismantled to make way for a new policy of multiculturalism that provided support to people from Southeast Asia seeking asylum from local conflicts. In the years that followed, Australia maintained an open but highly conservative approach to migration, but in 2001, following the September 11 attacks in the US, we moved to a discourse of high alert that was grounded in the War on Terror. Australia's response to people who arrived by boat had been strict, moving individuals to detention centres established in remote locations, but in 2001 we began a policy of turning back the boats and offshore processing in Nauru and Papua New Guinea (McDonnell, 2023). In 2012, offshore processing was expanded to ban all people who arrived by boat from being able to settle in Australia, regardless of their refugee application. Cementing this policy, the government ensured that the exclusion of asylum seekers was firmly embedded in a discourse of racism, distrust and othering. Over 4,000 people moved to offshore detention have been relocated to another country, but ten years on, 140 people remain in limbo. The significant negative impact of these policies on their physical and mental health is unjust and unfair (McDonnell, 2023).

Global context: The UK follows Australia's offshore model

Australia's model of offshore processing and detention for asylum seekers who arrive by boat has been sharply criticised by the UNHCR, but, despite this, some countries are seeking to emulate it. In 2022, the UK passed the Nationality and Borders Act, which criminalised asylum seekers, proposing their removal to a third country for offshore processing, and the pushing back of boats found in the English Channel. The legislation proposed the social exclusion of asylum seekers based on their method of arrival, modelling Australia's offshore processes which have been condemned by the UNHCR and criticised around the world as a system founded on the abuse of human rights (McDonnell, 2023).

Let's finish

Through this chapter we have carefully considered Australia's population, looking closely at who we are, how we live and our experiences of health and climate change. We identified many differences in health outcomes across different population groups and communities and considered these health inequities in relation to the social and political determinants of health, focusing specifically on the ways different forms of social exclusion undermine access and participation in our social, cultural, economic and political environments. Our consideration of the impact of politics and policy focused on key communities and identity groups including the LGBTIQA+ community and people living with disabilities. We also examined the roll-out of policies and political processes as they related to COVID-19 and migration policy and identified how the notion of community can be used positively but can also be used by political players to disempower and create division.

Summary

After reading this chapter, you should now be able to:

- Describe the notions of diversity, identity and community.
- Explore data describing Australia's diversity and critically analyse the experiences of health and climate change for different population groups.
- Critically analyse the social patterns of health and illness for people from different communities and identity groups in Australia.
- Define the notions of health inequity and social exclusion and critically analyse how policy and politics socially exclude different communities and identity groups.
- Critique the notion of identity politics and the processes used by policies and politics to create divisions between communities.

Tutorial exercises

1   Map the community where you live. Identify the key population groups, key health issues and local health and social care services available. What health inequities care you identify? Map out a plan that considers how you would use this information to advocate for better public health services and supports to meet the needs of your community?
2   Select a public health policy targeting a particular population group. Can you identify ways in which the policy is impacting positively and negative on your population group? Are there particular forms of social exclusion the policy is trying to address? Or do you think it will magnify experiences of social exclusion?
3   Identify a critical area of social exclusion impacting a particular population group. Design a policy response that will address the forms of social exclusion you have identified. What would the response look like and how might you pitch it to the health minister?

Further reading

ABS Community Profiles. Available at: https://www.abs.gov.au/census/guide-census-data/about-census-tools/community-profiles
Crenshaw, K. W. 2017. *On intersectionality: Essential writings*. New York: The New Press.
Every Australian Counts. Available at: www.everyaustraliancounts.com.au. (Disability advocacy site).
Friel, S. 2019. *Climate change and the people's health*. Oxford: Oxford University Press.
Friel, S., Collin, J., Daube, M., Depoux, A., Freudenberg, N., Gilmore, A. B., Johns, P., Laar, A., Marten, R., McKee, M., & Mialon, M. 2023. Commercial determinants of health: Future directions. *The Lancet*, 401(10383), 1229–1240.
Solar, O., & Irwin, A. 2010. A conceptual framework for action on the social determinants of health. Geneva: WHO Document Production Services.
UNHCR (UN High Commission for Refugees). Available at: www.unhcr.org.

References

ABS (Australian Bureau of Statistics). 2021. Snapshot of Australia. Available at: https://www.abs.gov.au/statistics/people/people-and-communities/snapshot-australia/2021 (accessed 21 June 2023).
AIHW (Australian Institute of Health and Welfare). 2021. Australia's welfare 2021: Data insights; snapshots and; in brief. Cat. no. AUS 236. Canberra: AIHW.

AIHW (Australian Institute of Health and Welfare). 2022. Australia's health 2022: Data insights; snapshots and; in brief. Canberra: AIHW. Badgett, M. L. 2011. Social inclusion and the value of marriage equality in Massachusetts and the Netherlands. *Journal of Social Issues*, 67(2), 316–334.

Bambra, C., Fox, D., & Scott-Samuel, A. 2005. Towards a politics of health. *Health Promotion International*, 20(2), 187–193. https://doi.org/10.1093/heapro/dah608.

Bretherton, I., Thrower, E., Zwickl, S., Wong, A., Chetcuti, D., Grossmann, M., ... & Cheung, A. S. 2021. The health and well-being of transgender Australians: A national community survey. *LGBT Health*, 8(1), 42–49. Carmona, E. 2018. Mojo Juju talks identity, Native Tongue and growing up with Pauline Hanson. Available at: https://fbiradio.com/mojo-juju-interview/ (accessed 24 June 2023).

Casey, L. J., Bowman, S. J., Wootton, B. M., McAloon, J., & Power, E. 2022. 'A tremendous outpouring of love and affection': A template analysis of positive experiences during a major LGBTQ rights campaign. *Journal of Homosexuality*, 1–23.

Chavis, D. M., & Lee, K. 2015. What is community anyway? *Stanford Social Innovation Review*. https://doi.org/10.48558/EJJ2-JJ82.

Crooks, K., Casey, D., & Ward, J. S. 2020. First Nations peoples leading the way in COVID-19 pandemic planning, response and management. *Medical Journal of Australia*, 213(4), 151–152.

CSDH(Commission on Social Determinants of Health). 2008. Closing the gap in a generation: Health equity through action on the social determinants of health. Commission on Social Determinants of Health final report. Geneva: World Health Organization. Drabble, L. A., Wootton, A. R., Veldhuis, C. B., Riggle, E. D., Rostosky, S. S., Lannutti, P. J., Balsam, K. F. , & Hughes, T. L. 2021. Perceived psychosocial impacts of legalized same-sex marriage: A scoping review of sexual minority adults' experiences. *PloS One*, 16(5), e0249125.

Friel, S. 2020. Climate change and the people's health: The need to exit the consumptagenic system. *The Lancet*, 395(10225), 666–668.

Friel, S. 2022. Climate change, society, and health inequities. *The Medical Journal of Australia*, 217(9), 466.

Friel, S., Price, S., Goldman, S., Baum, F., Townsend, B., & Schram, A. 2021. Australian COVID-19 policy responses: A health equity report card. Canberra: Menzies Centre for Health Governance, School of Regulation and Global Governance, Australian National University.

Habibis, D. 2019. The illness experience: Lay perspectives, disability, and chronic illness. In J. Germov (ed.), *Second opinion: An introduction to health sociology* (6th edn). South Melbourne: Oxford University Press, pp. 261–269.

Hall, S., & Du Gay, P. (eds) 1996. *Questions of cultural identity*. London: Sage.

Klein, E. 2020. Australia has been stigmatising unemployed people for almost 100 years. COVID-19 is our big chance to change this. *The Conversation*.

Lowe, T. 2021. What is community and why is it important?Centre for Public Impact. Available at: https://www.centreforpublicimpact.org/insights/what-is-community-and-why-is-it-important (accessed 22 June 2023).

Lyons, K. 2022. Australia violated the rights of Torres Strait Islanders by failing to act on climate change, the UN says. Here's what that means. *The Conversation*.

Marmot, M., & Wilkinson, R. 2005. Poverty, social exclusion, and minorities, in M. Marmot & R. Wilkinson (eds), *Social determinants of health* (2nd edn). Oxford: Oxford Academic.

McDonnell, E. 2023. UK joins global race to the bottom on migration importing Australia's deadly policies. *Asylum Insights*. Available at: https://www.asyluminsight.com/mcdonnell. (accessed 22 June 2023).

Okoli, A. C. 2003. Introduction to the special issue – identity: Now you don't see it; now you do. *Identity: An International Journal of Theory and Research*, 3(1), 1–7.

Shannon, B., & Smith, S. J. 2017. Dogma before diversity: The contradictory rhetoric of controversy and diversity in the politicisation of Australian queer-affirming learning materials. *Sex Education*, 17(3), 242–255.

Solar, O., & Irwin, A. 2010. A conceptual framework for action on the social determinants of health. Geneva: WHO Document Production Services.

UNHCR. 2023. *Global trends: Forced displacement in 2022*. Geneva:UNHCR.

White, P. 1998. Urban life and social stress. In D. Pinder (ed.), *The new Europe: Economy, society and environment*. Chichester: Wiley.

Williamson, B. 2021. The COVID-19 crisis in western NSW Aboriginal communities is a nightmare realised. *The Conversation*.

Zevallos, Z. 2011. What is Otherness? *The Other Sociologist*, 14 October. Available at: https://otherso ciologist.com/otherness-resources/

Podcasts

ABC Listen. Let us in – podcast series on the experiences of people with disabilities featuring Kurt Fearnley and Sarah Shands.

Policy Forum Net. A vision for a healthy Australia featuring Sharon Friels.

Part II
Political Determinants of Our Lives

3 Housing and Energy

Stefanie Plage and Rose-Marie Stambe

> A decent life was the train that hadn't hit you, the slumlord you hadn't offended, the malaria you hadn't caught.
>
> (Katherine Boo, 2012, *Behind the Beautiful Forevers*)

Learning objectives

After studying this chapter, you should be able to:

1 Understand how political factors affect the health of individuals and communities via differential access to appropriate housing and sustainable sources of energy.
2 Analyse the dynamics between negative health impacts of poor housing and energy infrastructures, and the socio-political landscapes they are embedded in.
3 Assess the logics underpinning housing and energy policy decisions in their repercussions for the health of different demographics within various geopolitical contexts.
4 Critique the economic rationalities informing monetary and fiscal solutions to housing and energy issues from a political determinants of health perspective.
5 Propose alternative conceptual frameworks to address the pressing need to meet the energy and housing needs in all communities on a planetary scale.

Snapshot

Housing is one of the most fundamental needs all people have in common. A place to call home is more than a roof that offers protection from the elements: it provides a secure base from which to pursue daily activities and personal goals. Despite the universal nature of the need to be housed, opportunities to live safely and comfortably are unequally distributed across the world. In 2018, about 24% of the urban population, that is, over 1 billion people lived in slums (UN, 2021). The opening quote for this chapter is taken from Katherine Boo's (2012) book, *Behind the Beautiful Forevers*, detailing life in a Mumbai slum. It captures the serendipity of survival, defying the individualistic faith in our capacity to forge our own destinies. Access to clean water and food, safe communities, education, privacy, and dignity are highly politicized. Local political actors as well as global agencies are stakeholders in competing agendas, into which the people most affected by these dynamics have little input. The COVID-19 pandemic has made this even more tangible. Directions to self-isolate and implement strict sanitation regimes fall flat in overcrowded spaces with poor energy infrastructure. Lockdowns and orders to return 'home' issued to migrant workers – often violently enforced

DOI: 10.4324/9781003315490-7

by state and local governments – disproportionately affected the urban poor who subsist through informal economic activities. As environmental degradation proliferates, we will likely see more disasters, including the pandemic spread of infectious diseases, but also weather events and conflicts over scarce resources. While the world's poor continue to feel repercussions most acutely, these challenges affect the health of all countries and communities across the globe.

Let's begin

Housing, energy, and health are embedded in planetary relations of supply and demand, migration and labour, urbanization, and globalization. This chapter traces housing and energy as interrelated political determinants of health primarily in the Australian context but always in dialogue with extant dynamics in other parts of the world. We begin by fleshing out the factors that affect housing policies and practice, before turning to dynamics around energy. The first section of this chapter outlines the socio-political context of housing affordability and the consequences of poor housing conditions for the health of individuals and communities. We then discuss homelessness as a phenomenon in which political determinants of health eventuate with often catastrophic and long-lasting health repercussions. We also situate housing within debates on meanings and values and critically engage with contemporary policy solutions to housing issues. This section concludes by juxtaposing the health and livelihoods of the urban poor in megacities, and Indigenous people and communities in Australia. The second section of this chapter outlines the health implications of energy policies and practices. We tease out the health effects of rising energy costs and poor building standards, before discussing global politics around environmental degradation. We engage with supranational approaches to just energy transitions and introduce various stakeholders in energy as a political determinant of health. The chapter concludes with a summary of key points highlighting the interconnectedness of housing and energy issues.

The health impacts of the politics of housing and housing policy

Housing

Access to quality and affordable housing is a perennial issue for housing policy and practice that is not restricted to the Global South. Countries in the Americas, Europe and Oceania likewise struggle to provide accessible housing for their populations. Take Australia, one of the wealthier nations in the world, as an example. Anglicare Australia conducts yearly snapshots to assess rental affordability across the country. They use the idea of housing stress to measure affordability. For low-income groups, housing stress is present, when 30% or more of the household's budget is put towards paying rent (Anglicare, 2022). In other words, a rental listing is considered unaffordable for a person or a family if it exceeds this benchmark. On 19 March 2022, Anglicare surveyed more than 45,000 rental listings and found that only one of them would have been affordable for a single person over the age of 18 living on Youth Allowance. The prospect for other household types was similarly bleak, with 0–1.4% of rental listings being affordable for households on different types of government benefits. For household types relying on minimum wage, this proportion ranged between 0.7% and 15.3%.

The policy response to the housing affordability crisis focuses on the price of housing. Then-Reserve Bank of Australia governor, Philip Lowe is quoted as saying (Hutchens & Whitson, 2023):

The way that this ends up fixing itself, unfortunately, is through higher housing prices and higher rents … The increase in supply can't happen immediately, but higher prices do lead people to economise on housing. That's the price mechanism at work. We need more people on average to live in each dwelling, and prices do that.

Monetary and fiscal policy decisions (e.g., changes to interest rates and tax rules) informed by this logic conceive of greater occupancy rates in the available housing stock as a solution to insufficient supply. Yet, it is well known that many social and public housing estates already suffer from overcrowding. Overcrowding is one the biggest known drivers of homelessness among Indigenous people in the Northern Territory, where the last Census showed a homelessness rate of nearly 5% (Roussos, 2023). Social and public housing are often a last resort for people who cannot afford a rental unit in the private market. Applicants for social housing are waitlisted and depending on where they live and their ability to demonstrate need, might not be offered a place to live for years.

Political factors also affect the quality of housing. In some European countries, for example, Germany, the private rental market features legal protections for tenants that enable greater stability in their tenancy and provide leverage to have properties well maintained. This has significant benefits for tenant health and wellbeing. Unaddressed water leaks in poorly ventilated buildings can lead to mould that worsens allergies and other health concerns. Young children are vulnerable to respiratory infections and asthmatic exacerbations due to living in damp environments, often with complications that can affect them over the life course. Likewise, fixed-term lease agreements resulting in frequent moves can impact healthy development. Moving houses can disrupt belonging and interfere with the cultivation of social support networks. Residential mobility is associated with short term academic, social and emotional issues in child development. What is more, few properties cater to the needs of aging citizens and people with disabilities. Housing accessibility comprises modifying a property to meet an occupant's individual needs and enable independent living. Where housing affordability and stock are low, there is little incentive for landlords to invest in their properties to make them accessible.

These dynamics are further complicated by the interrelated types of meanings and values assigned to housing, land, and home. Housing has become defined as a private investment rather than a public good. Property owners are considered to have a reasonable expectation to receive financial gain from their investment, and tax mechanisms such as 'negative gearing' provide some protection from losses in Australia. For example, if the expenses for a property are greater than the gains from renting it out, the resulting costs can be offset from other taxable income. The commodification of housing informs a policy logic in which stimulation of the private market rather than increasing the public housing stock is the primary mechanism to expand housing supply. Many countries, including Australia, are now experiencing the failure of past governments to develop public housing over the long term, as the spread of extreme poverty and housing instability in their communities.

Limelight: Treatment First or Housing First?

There are two broad policies originating in the USA aimed at solving chronic homelessness: 'Treatment First' (TF) and 'Housing First' (HF). TF has dominated in the past, approaching homelessness as associated with a person's lifestyle. Informed by the tenet of individual responsibility, TF understands homelessness as driven by undesirable and often medicalized behaviours (i.e., use of drugs or violence). TF interventions seek to address these behaviours to make people ready for housing. HF is a paradigmatic shift responding to the failure of TF to end chronic homelessness. HF pays greater attention to housing as a social determinant of health. HF implements permanent supportive housing that integrates other forms of care for people experiencing chronic homelessness. Housing allocation is based on vulnerability assessments to house those first whose health is most compromised: housing itself becomes a form of health care. There is a growing evidence base that supports the HF approach when it comes to housing outcomes and cost savings for the public purse. HF's permanent supportive housing model has proliferated and seen many manifestations beyond the USA. Today's debates focus largely on balancing the fidelity to HF principles (e.g., permanence and harm minimization) with adaptation to fit local contexts (see Padgett, Henwood & Tsemberis, 2016).

Homelessness

Insecure housing is a critical social problem disproportionately affecting people with low incomes or past experiences of homelessness. Recent data indicates a worsening of the issue in developed countries. In the USA, homelessness increased by 2% between 2019 and 2020, reversing the decline in homelessness observed in the prior decade (NAEH, 2022). Data from 36 countries on the number of people reported as homeless by the public housing authorities and collated in the OECD's Affordable Housing Database, shows declines in the homelessness rate in some countries, but increases in several others (OECD, 2021). In Australia, the number of people experiencing homelessness between 2018 and 2022 grew at double the rate of the national population (Pawson et al., 2022).

People with experience of homelessness live less healthy and shorter lives. Higher incidence and prevalence of acute and chronic conditions among homeless populations include cardiovascular disease and cancer, mental ill-health, injury, respiratory illness, HIV/AIDS, sexual ill-health, and infectious diseases. Access barriers to health services result in unmet needs including for reproductive health care, foot care, dental care, care after hospital discharge, mental health and primary care. Experiences of health and illness are shaped by the political determinants that prevail in a local context. In the USA, barriers are often financial in nature given a complex and patchy health insurance system. However, the cost of healthcare is only part of the picture. In Australia, Medicare as a tax-funded health scheme is intended to provide basic health services to all citizens in need, yet, health inequities persist. The reasons for that lie in a complicated mix of individual and structural level determinants, including stigma, health-seeking behaviours and health services configurations. Allowing homelessness as a phenomenon to persist in itself is a political determinant of (ill) health that perpetuates and normalizes the regular exclusion of a portion of the population from the most taken-for-granted salutogenic practices and resources (Plage & Parsell, 2022). Shelter protects from heat, cold and rain, provides access to hygiene facilities and safety from violence. The experience of extreme poverty also diminishes opportunities to pursue healthy nutrition, physical activity, sleep and rest routines. To meet their basic needs, people often rely on charitable organizations which have taken over responsibilities from the government to care for the most disadvantaged in advanced welfare states.

Tackling homelessness is made more complicated by the fact that what is even considered a home – and by extension who is considered homeless – differs greatly across countries. Slum dwellers on the fringes of the world's megacities often share shelter that is overcrowded, without access to clean water or sanitation, electricity or other amenities, yet they are captured and counted in their own statistics. Across developed countries, definitions of what homelessness is are not universal either. Whether one is considered homeless may take into account if the person has a disability, is able to exercise control over their environment, or the presence of domains that comprise a home. Modalities of homelessness are also transforming and are not always readily recognizable as such. Street living, marked by rough sleeping, now only makes up a small percentage of people who are experiencing homelessness, with many more people living in overcrowded dwellings, cars, caravans, tents, boarding houses or staying with friends or family for as long as they are welcome. There are also changes in the demographic profile of people experiencing homelessness in Australia and elsewhere. Women over the age of 55 are among the fastest-growing cohorts of people becoming newly homeless. They feel let down by states, communities, and families on their paths into homelessness (Goodall et al., 2022). Notably, becoming homeless intersects with gender, age, ethnicity, race, and migration as social determinants to affect platform workers, international students and Indigenous and older people disproportionately. The changes in who is affected by homelessness and how homelessness is experienced across different demographics necessitate tailored policy responses that have to contend with a gamut of social issues, such as domestic and family violence, exploitative and unregulated informal labour markets, cultural understandings of housing as a commodity rather than a public good, ageism, ableism, racism, colonialism, and many other issues. In housing as a political determinant of health coalesce historical and contemporary injustices that can only be effectively remedied if recognized and addressed comprehensively.

Spotlight: Policy process

COVID-19 responses to homelessness

How policymakers respond to issues of housing and homelessness very much depends on how the problem is framed in the first place, or as policy analyst Carol Bacchi (2009) asks: *What is the problem represented to be?* In their article, Cameron Parsell, Andrew Clarke and Ella Kuskoff (2023) analyse the dramatic change in how policies address homelessness. They contrast a poverty of ambition to end homelessness in countries such as Australia, the UK, the USA, and much of Europe preceding the COVID-19 pandemic, with unprecedented interventions and expenditure to house the homeless in unused hospitality and student accommodation following its onset. They argue, this is not only evidence of the capacity to solve homelessness as a matter of political will, but they also explain this shift as a function of how people experiencing homelessness became reframed as both *at risk* from contracting COVID-19 and *a threat* to the health of the non-homeless population if left unhoused and free to transmit the virus.

Let's do

What is the (housing) problem represented to be? Work in small groups. Identify which government agency holds the housing portfolio in your country or state. Locate two documents that outline policy principles, strategic plans, goals, as well as outcome measures. Discuss how housing is framed in policy and practice. Can you glimpse from this exercise what the problem with housing is represented to be?

Spotlight: Advocacy Action

Health Home Hope

As part of a research study on housing and health in Queensland, Australia, participants with lived experience of homelessness were asked to use photographs to tell the story of what health looks and feels like and what it means to them. This approach follows in the footsteps of community-based participatory action research using photovoice to reach policymakers and strengthen advocacy. The photographs were curated into an exhibition and put on public display (Plage et al., 2023) (Figure 3.1). Some 60 guests attended the launch, including contributors with lived experience of homelessness, local politicians and key stakeholders from government and non-government organizations active in the housing and social care sector where the project was carried out. The lively discussions on the night exemplify the potential for reimagining housing and health as something that is done within socio-political relations of care.

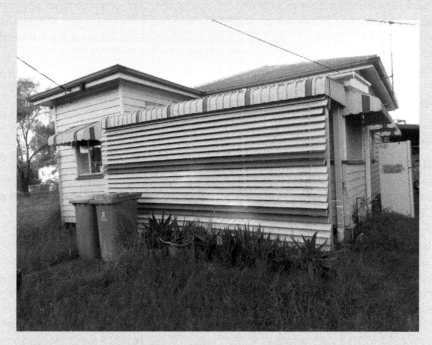

Figure 3.1 MY HOME. My safe place. Nobody can get me here.
Source: Caption and photograph by Jessie Morwood (Plage et al., 2023). Reproduced with permission.

Urbanization

Beyond housing affordability and homelessness, where and how we live together in communities greatly affect our opportunities for good health. Societies have become urbanized with large parts of many countries' populations concentrated in urban centres. There are now dozens of megacities globally, each of them home to more than 10 million people. In megacities, space comes at a premium and the distinction between public and private spaces is often blurred. Lata Lutfun Nahar (2021) explores the lack of available job opportunities in the formal sector and financial resources in Dhaka, a megacity in Bangladesh. Urban poor rely on access to public space for their livelihoods. However, city officials are invested in demonstrating that their city has earned its rightful place in the modern global community. The visibility of abject poverty and informal economic activities is perceived as incongruent with an image of progressive urbanism. In turn, the urban poor become displaced from public spaces, effectively denying them a right to the city. Once more we are reminded of the epigraph at the beginning of this chapter, capturing the sense of fatefulness of survival in a megacity's slum. Policy narratives emphasize education, skills, and entrepreneurial ingenuity as a way out of poverty, not only in developing countries. We are all too familiar with the 'rags to riches' narrative that promises rewards for hard work, which illustrates how we think about individuals' agency over their lives. Of course, this way of approaching social mobility neglects the structural and political constraints which we all face when pursuing aspirations for a better life. The flipside of the 'rags to riches' narrative is that we more readily believe that billionaires have earned their fortunes (e.g., by taking risks and applying themselves) and that the poor are to blame for their misery. Explanations of social disadvantage favour individual responsibility rather than account for political determinants.

Global context: Sustainable Development Goal 11

You have come across the UN Sustainable Development Goals (SDGs) in other chapters. Remember that SDGs articulate policy objectives for the global community, coupled with a target that allows us to track progress towards meeting these objectives. Sustainable Development Goal 11 seeks to 'Make cities inclusive, safe, resilient and sustainable'. The UN elaborates on SDG 11:

> [The] challenges cities face can be overcome in ways that allow them to continue to thrive and grow, while improving resource use and reducing pollution and poverty. The future we want includes cities of opportunities for all, with access to basic services, energy, housing, transportation and more.

There are a number of targets that outline when and how this vision for the future is to be made reality. For our purposes, Target 11.1 is particularly salient: 'By 2030, ensure access for all to adequate, safe and affordable housing and basic services and upgrade slums.' At present, it is doubtful whether this milestone will be met within the allotted time frame. Nonetheless, SDGs fulfil an important function in holding global and local governance accountable, prompting critical revisions to the political determinants of health.

Let's refresh

Revisit the passages in this book outlining the UN SDGs, their purpose, and mechanisms. In small groups, map the various factors that contribute to the complexities in progressing towards meeting SDG 11. Draw lines to visualize their interconnectedness. Can you identify other SDGs that are salient to the planetary housing and energy agenda?

While remote communities far from urban centres with small population sizes face vastly different challenges than urban poor in megacities, we can observe some similar rationalities at work in health promotion campaigns in these settings, particularly those implemented with Indigenous communities. Indigenous communities in Australia and First Nations elsewhere have been targeted by political projects framed as health intervention since the beginning of European colonial expansion. Often racialized interventions have focused on controlling Indigenous populations via health governance aimed at discrete issues, for example, contagious disease, gambling, alcoholism, smoking, obesity, drug use and many others (see Nicoll, 2012). In recent history, government policies focusing on the harms to individuals and communities stemming from alcohol consumption illustrate this point. Such policies have entailed interventionist strategies that make it harder for people to buy and drink alcohol, for example, by banning or highly regulating the sale of alcoholic beverages within a certain geographical radius and punishing the violation of such prohibitionist rules. Punitive strategies illustrate how health promotion can become a form of control, often with little consideration of local political actors or community preferences. Recent interventions, often labelled 'Indigenous-led', seek to address alcohol-induced harms by establishing 'dry communities'. The successes of such interventions in reducing alcohol-related injury and hospitalizations are mixed, with some programmes evidently working, and others producing non-findings or ambivalent evidence. Importantly, a policy focus on curbing individual alcohol consumption among Indigenous people in remote communities suggests that identifying as Indigenous constitutes a risk factor. Statistically, however, Indigenous Australians are less likely to drink alcohol than other Australians (Australian Government, Department of Health and Aged Care, n.d.).

The focus on individualized and pathologized behaviours, such as alcohol consumption, forms another piece of the puzzle in explaining the social disadvantage experienced by Indigenous people, without attending to the failure to integrate Indigenous knowledge and practices into local and global political systems or redress the repercussions of discrimination and institutional racism as the perpetuation of historical injustices. These rationalities also continue the allocation of certain spaces and places to Indigenous peoples. Marcia Langton (1981) critiqued the tendency to align 'urban' with 'white' and 'rural' with 'Aboriginal'. In Australia's urban centres, many Indigenous people are affected by a trend towards gentrification. Driven by real estate interests, neighbourhoods near inner cities and central business districts that used to be inhabited by people with low socioeconomic status, often from Indigenous or culturally and racially marginalized backgrounds, are becoming lifestyle suburbs. Gentrified neighbourhoods attract investors and wealthy residents who seek bespoke opportunities for cultural consumption (i.e., coffee shops, music theatres, specialized grocery stores). Gentrification has the potential to displace those who previously have called these suburbs home, because they are no longer able to afford to live there or to participate in public life. Shifts in neighbourhood demographic profile can be accompanied by diminishing other opportunities for equitable lives, for example, proximity to a good school or a health clinic with comprehensive services. Poorer neighbourhoods are more likely to experience a lack of resources to promote positive health, such as recreational facilities and green spaces, or even night-time ambience conducive to rest and sleep.

Health outcomes differ on markers, such as life expectancy, all-cause mortality and morbidity, depending on where people live, but also across populations with Indigenous, European, and other settler ancestry. Access to health is better in urban centres and improving the opportunities for good health of all, including residents in remote communities, is a formidable challenge for policy and practice that requires the transformation of collective practices, and reimagining health governance beyond the cultivation of control and individual responsibility.

Indigenous perspective: Health promotion: Deadly Choices

An ethnography of social networking sites undertaken by a non-Indigenous researcher in partnership with an Indigenous community-controlled health organization, and a team of Indigenous and non-Indigenous supervisors, advisors, critical friends, and mentors explored opportunities for health promotion agendas to foster self-determination and empowerment in an Indigenous Australian context (McPhail-Bell et al., 2018). The Deadly Choices programme is an Indigenous-led health promotion initiative underpinned by five principles: (1) the creation of dialogue; (2) the building of community online and offline; (3) the incentivization of healthy online engagement; (4) the celebration of Indigenous identity and culture; and (5) the prioritization of partnerships. The study argued that adherence to these principles shifted power from health promotion practitioners to Indigenous people and communities. Transferring Deadly Choices principles to social networking sites used by mainstream health promotion practice can facilitate respect and support for Indigenous self-determination.

Let's do

Governments can support people's health with targeted urban planning. For example, managing urban sprawl and enhancing mixed-use zoning (i.e., the co-location of residential, educational, and business spaces) can reduce commuting and pollution, and increase incidental exercise and healthy physical activity. Imagine your local town planning office asked for a briefing paper aimed at modifying your city to make it a healthier place to live. List three suggestions and give a compelling rationale on why the town planners should implement them.

The health impacts of the politics of energy and energy policy

Energy bills

The rising costs of energy bills have become a critical issue for Australian individuals and families. The escalating costs of energy bills have substantial implications for public health, particularly in terms of access to basic needs, such as heating, cooling, and lighting. High energy bills have a detrimental impact on physical and mental health, and are disproportionately burdensome for low-income households and vulnerable populations. This section aims to explore the multifaceted ways in which high energy bills impact health, emphasizing the unique challenges faced in Australia.

Concern about the rising cost of energy bills is not a recent phenomenon, but the dramatic impact of the COVID-19 pandemic and geopolitical concerns, like the Ukrainian conflict, have meant that the price of energy for Australians has increased significantly and will continue to do so. In March 2023, the Australian Energy Regulator (AER) – the main organization that manages wholesale electricity and gas markets across Australia – flagged a 24% increase on energy bills. The Victorian Regulator (i.e., the Essential Services Commission), even predicted a 30% increase. While the transition to renewable energies could provide a relief, that is a long-term plan that requires more investment in transmission and energy storage. In the interim, many Australians are already struggling with the cost-of-living crisis in 2023, and will also be further affected by a sharp increase in energy prices.

A key concern about the rising costs of energy is that it will create energy poverty. Energy poverty is the inability to afford adequate energy service or the need to reduce the energy consumption of a household in such a way that it has a negative effect on the health and wellbeing of the residents. Planetary climate change will increase temperature-related deaths, and this is a particular concern for Australia. In Australia, low-income households often face difficulties in meeting energy costs, leading to inadequate heating or cooling and increased vulnerability to temperature-related illnesses. This is especially an issue in Australia's heatwaves. Heat stress can exacerbate existing conditions and older people are most vulnerable to its effects. Hyperthermia also leads to a lack of concentration and fatigue (Hanna, 2020). Research from the USA suggests that as planetary heatwaves become more frequent, there will also be an increase in deaths from injury due to the impact of extreme heat to increase conflict and interpersonal violence. Internationally, regions with extreme climates experience similar challenges, for example, in the UK, the inability to pay for energy bills means that 9,700 deaths are caused by living in a cold home, which is about the same as the number of people who die from breast or prostate cancer in the UK over a year (Guertler & Smith, 2018). The cost of energy also has implications for mental health. The financial strain caused by high energy bills can lead to psychological distress and exacerbate existing mental health conditions. Stress, anxiety, and depression have been associated with energy bill-related financial hardship, as individuals and families struggle to maintain a comfortable living environment. Such mental health impacts are observed across various socio-economic groups and underscore the importance of affordable energy access.

The impact of high energy bills is nonetheless greatest for vulnerable populations such as low-income households, the elderly, and individuals with chronic illnesses. Disadvantaged communities across national contexts are more likely to experience health disparities resulting from unaffordable energy bills, perpetuating existing inequalities. In Australia, for instance, Aboriginal and Torres Strait Islanders often face energy poverty due to remote living conditions and limited access to affordable energy options. The urgency of planetary climate action has meant some governments, such as the Queensland Government, in the Queensland Energy and Jobs Plan, have prioritized energy justice for disadvantaged people, especially Aboriginal Torres Strait Islanders.

Addressing the health impacts of high energy bills requires a comprehensive approach involving policymakers, health care professionals and community organizations. The impacts cited above shed light on the urgency of addressing the cost of energy beyond the political cycle. In its latest budget (2023–2024), the Federal Government promised to focus on the cost-of-living crisis. The budget includes up to $3 billion of electricity bill relief for eligible households and small businesses, alongside a rebate of up to $500 for households and $650 for small businesses. Federal and state governments will also offer $500 relief for pensioners, veterans, and recipients of other support payments. A Household Energy Upgrades Fund will hold $1.3 billion for low-cost loans to double-glaze windows, and install solar panels. Another $300 million has been set aside for states to invest in energy upgrades to social housing. In addition to these short-term incentives, other policies are needed to transition to renewables and support a more reasonable cost of energy to ensure energy justice.

Energy ratings

Energy ratings are designed to assess and communicate energy efficiency of a product, or in the case of a building, the structure. Energy ratings can be used to inform health promotion alongside their stated purpose, which is to reduce energy consumption and greenhouse gas emission. This is particularly pertinent when we consider the design of a house and building as part of their energy ratings. Energy-inefficient housing poses health risks, such as mould growth, indoor air pollution, and inadequate ventilation. These conditions can lead to respiratory illnesses, allergies, and other health complications. These issues are more prevalent in socio-economically disadvantaged areas, underscoring the need for energy-efficient policies and affordable housing solutions. Considering we spend up to 70% of our time in our home, we need to take seriously the health risks of living in an unhealthy home environment (Baker et al., 2019). The Property Council suggests that every house should have an energy star rating, and this would support a reduction in planetary greenhouse emission from properties. It would also mean that buyers and renters are able to contribute to climate action. Currently, there is a National House Energy rating scheme that is used for new buildings but could be extended to a National Construction code for new houses to meet minimum standards. A key problem in this area for Australia is the lack of sufficient data on the energy efficiency of our existing housing, which makes developing evidence-based policy more challenging. The International Energy Agency recommends that advanced economies should endorse a net zero-ready building code. The focus of this section is to look at the potential health implications and the need for a more holistic understanding of energy ratings and building design.

Spotlight: Policy process: just transitions

Just transitions prioritize equitable outcomes for workers and communities during shifts to sustainable economies. These transitions address social, economic, and environmental challenges associated with moving away from carbon-intensive industries. The term originated in the 1970s when unions raised concerns about the impact of environmental regulations on workers' rights and health. Just transitions advocate for phasing out polluting industries and adopting cleaner alternatives. Yet, there is still debate about their meaning, political support, and beneficiaries. Coal workers and their communities have often felt excluded from the decision-making process during 'just' transitions. Australia and other countries are rapidly transitioning to renewables, but the inclusion of just transition principles in policies varies. Colorado, the Netherlands, and Poland have explicitly endorsed just transitions, while others, like Australia, have not. Considering social justice in transitions, particularly for marginalized communities, is crucial. Planetary just transitions, as advocated by scholars like Dimitris Stevis, aim to benefit both advanced and developing economies. Policy development in this area is evolving, and incorporating community voices will lead to better and fairer outcomes.

One key area to consider when developing building energy ratings is air ventilation. There are few rules for ventilation, and the Australian construction code does allow for buildings to be constructed to hold many people, like a nightclub with 1000 people, with no ventilation. Considering the health impacts, more work needs to be done in this area. The *Air Quality Handbook* was sent out for consultation in 2022, in response to the COVID-19 pandemic and the greater awareness of how airborne viruses can spread, and the importance of good indoor air quality and ventilation. Better building standards that cover the upper limits for all contaminants ensure standards of air quality with important health impacts (Hanmer, 2022).

The quality of housing depends on socio-economic status. In places like Australia, there are no regulations for obtaining a building permit to build in some regional and remote Indigenous communities in the Northern Territory. This means that houses can be poorly constructed, are uninsulated, and have inadequate plumbing and no air conditioners. If people have pre-existing health conditions, the poor standard of housing in the heat can exacerbate their conditions. This means that some people are living in effective hot boxes that detrimentally affect their health. Temperature plays a crucial role in maintaining occupants' health and comfort. Disadvantaged groups are particularly susceptible to the negative health effects that arise from living in homes with inadequate temperature conditions. Social housing units with insufficient insulation, poor heating or cooling systems, and inadequate temperature control can expose residents to extreme temperatures, leading to adverse health effects. Heat-related illnesses, such as heat exhaustion and heatstroke, are prevalent in buildings with inadequate cooling systems, while cold temperatures contribute to respiratory problems, cardiovascular issues, and increased susceptibility to infections. A recent study examined the temperature conditions within social housing in Australia, investigated the experiences of tenants, and considered potential options for improvement (Sansom et al., 2023). On average, participants experienced temperatures outside the recommended guidelines set by the World Health Organization (18–24°C) for 35% of the study period. Most participants expressed feeling cold or very cold during colder weather, and many found energy costs to be unaffordable. Building conditions emerged as a significant concern for participants, specifically issues, such as poor window and door sealing, lack of insulation, and inadequate space heating equipment. The study emphasized that implementing energy-efficient measures, such as draft sealing and insulation could greatly enhance the quality of their homes and living conditions.

There needs to be better energy efficiency for both new and older homes. There are new efficiency standards aiming for all new residential property to achieve a 7/10 star rating. To make this achievable, passive design can help, so too can double or triple glazing or having internal doors to close off rooms when not in use. Retrofitting older homes must be a key initiative in Australia, where homes built before the 1990s can have a very low rating, sometimes as low as 1 or 2/10. There are 10 million homes like this in Australia, meaning codes to improve new housing are not enough to ensure that the ecological footprint is reduced. Retrofitting can be more cost-effective than demolishing and rebuilding new homes, and more incentives should be in place not just for existing home occupiers but also for landlords to ensure a better spread of retrofit across the country. This should be a key policy agenda for Australia to improve planetary impact and climate action, as well as improving people's health.

Limelight: Voices from the Pacific Islands

Environmental leaders are cautiously optimistic about a nuclear fusion breakthrough that could lead to clean energy. Nuclear fusion does not emit greenhouse gases nor produce radioactive waste: it is the same process that powers the sun and the stars. Nuclear fusion technology is very promising for an endless supply of green energy, however, the technology itself is a long way off, and it could be decades before it can be deployed in the Pacific Islands. Private sector investment could speed up the process but not enough to meet global greenhouse targets. Nuclear science has left a tragic legacy in the Pacific. Some islands were used for nuclear bomb testing by the UK, the USA and France, leading to radiation. Communities are still dealing with the ongoing impact today. Further, Pacific Islands will be hardest hit by climate change, with rising sea levels shrinking land mass. The leaders representing Pacific Islands have voiced their concerns about countries not acting fast enough or taking technology like nuclear fusion seriously, even though it is safe. The plight of the Pacific Islands highlights how concerns about climate change are a planetary concern, and it requires multilevel and multi-country action and collaboration, especially for those countries that contributed less to carbon emissions and yet are still facing catastrophe without urgent and extraordinary worldwide action.

Deforestation

Deforestation, the widespread clearing of forests for various purposes, has profound health implications that affect both human and environmental well-being. In Queensland during 2018–2019, 680,000 hectares of habitat were destroyed, which is more than in the previous 18 years. In Brazil, 2.90 million hectares of natural forest were lost, according to Global Forest Watch (n.d.) – equivalent to 1.7 gross tonnage of greenhouse gas emissions. In both Queensland and Brazil, deforestation and land clearing take place to pursue economic interests, for example, to feed livestock. These staggering figures highlight the impact of deforestation. There are several aspects to consider when assessing how large-scale planetary deforestation impacts on people's health. This section teases out the health implications of planetary deforestation, highlighting its impact on air quality, water resources, infectious diseases, and human health.

The first aspect to consider is the impact that deforestation has on air quality. With the loss of trees, there is an increase in greenhouse gas emissions, leading to climate change and air pollution. Deforestation contributes to the release of vast amounts of carbon dioxide, which is a primary greenhouse gas responsible for global warming. This is most significant when deforestation is progressed using fire. In Brazil, research from the Human Rights Watch has highlighted how deforestation-related fires led to 2,195 hospitalizations for respiratory illnesses in 2019. This number only captures a fraction of the effects because social disadvantage impedes access to health care facilities. In other words, more people were adversely affected than the figures demonstrate, and, importantly, may not have received adequate medical care. The impact of deforestation on air quality is not just about direct effects on people's health, but also exemplifies the intersectionality of planetary climate change, human action against the environment, and the uneven distribution of wealth and resources in different societies.

Let's do

Go to the Global Forest Watch website and find the link for the Interactive Forest Map. Click on the option to analyse historical trends. Pick two places, one in the Global North and one in the Global South. Look at the trends over the past 20–30 years. Examine similarities and differences between the locations. How much forest has been lost? In what part of the country? What are the socio-demographics of the country in general, but also the locations where most of the deforestation has happened? What are the implications: (1) for the environment; (2) for society; and (3) for health? Bring together these insights into a comparative analysis on how deforestation impacts health in similar and different ways depending on the social context.

Deforestation also impacts water resources, including rivers, lakes, and groundwater. Forests act as natural water filters, absorbing rainfall and releasing it gradually, preventing soil erosion and maintaining the water table. Intact woodlands and forests protect soils and riverbanks – without them, water runs off, causing soil erosion and sedimentation. The River Nile runs through or along the border of 10 countries in North-East Africa. Its water flows have been greatly reduced from deforestation in the west of the continent. Rivers like the Nile are important resources: 200–300 million people rely on the river for their livelihood. Alteration in water systems can also reduce water quality, increase flooding, and spread waterborne diseases. Contaminated waters harbour pathogens and pollutants, leading to illnesses such as diarrhoea, cholera, and parasitic infections, particularly in communities relying on these sources for their daily needs. Research in Malawi, East Africa, has shown that deforestation has decreased locals' access to clean drinking water, with a 1.0 percentage point increase in deforestation leading to 0.93 percentage point decrease in access to clean drinking water (Mapulanga & Naito, 2019). Considering the considerable socio-economic disadvantage in Malawi means the decrease in access to clean water has an enormous impact on people's lives and their health.

Deforestation also plays a role in the spread of infectious diseases. Forest ecosystems provide habitats for diverse wildlife, including various disease-carrying vector species such as mosquitoes, ticks, and rodents. When forests are cleared, these species lose their natural habitats, forcing them to seek alternative hosts: this is how viruses jump from wildlife to humans. Deforestation causes a disruption in ecosystems and increases the contact and proximity of humans and wildlife, facilitating the transmission of zoonotic diseases, such as malaria, dengue fever, Lyme disease, and Ebola. The COVID-19 pandemic has brought this issue into focus at a planetary level. Its suspected origin in bats led to the global spread of the virus. Other diseases have been connected to deforestation, such as Ebola, Venezuelan equine encephalitis, and malaria. Yellow fever is another example. The virus that causes yellow fever lives in monkeys and is spread by mosquitoes. A yellow fever outbreak occurred in Kerio Valley Kenya, after deforestation had been taking place in the early 1990s. This was the first occurrence of the disease in this area (Tucker et al., 2017). Recognizing the importance of forests as essential ecosystems is crucial for maintaining a healthy planet and population. By taking proactive measures to curb deforestation and promote sustainable practices, we can strive towards a healthier future.

Indigenous perspective: Connection to Country

The connection to Country is of immense importance for Australian Aboriginal and Torres Strait Islander peoples and significantly impacts their health and wellbeing. Land is intertwined with cultural identity, spirituality, and traditional practices. Disruption of this connection has detrimental effects on health outcomes. Being connected to Country has been used to support people with dementia. First Nations are three to five times more likely to develop dementia and finding culturally appropriate ways to communicate and keep connected to Country is crucial to support high-level care. Additionally, 9.6 out of 1000 Aboriginal and Torres Strait Islander babies are stillborn or die within the first 28 days of life. Supporting mothers to birth on Country or find ways to connect to Country in a hospital setting, has been shown to support women having better outcomes, including the mother's sense of wellbeing. More recognition needs to be given for the Indigenous-led efforts to care for Country and address climate change. Indigenous peoples have been advocating for change and recognition of their knowledge of how to take care of the land, which became very prominent in the Australian Black Summer Fires of 2019–2020, but also in other areas, such as the sea (see https://youtu.be/Uu9V7waH5f0). Recognizing and respecting the importance of Country are crucial in promoting the health and wellbeing of Aboriginal and Torres Strait Islander peoples.

Let's think

China has been crippled by air pollution and is attempting to reduce its dependency on coal. The country has committed to shifting to renewable energies but is still a major burner of coal. In 2022, China invested $546 billion in renewables such as solar and wind energy and electric vehicles and batteries. This makes China the world leader in renewable energy expansion worldwide. There is also a push to quickly expand the Chinese electric vehicle market with current exports focused on Europe, with plans to export beyond. The cost of electric vehicles has dropped by 80% in the last 7 years. Individually or in groups, discuss what it means for China to be a world leader in electric vehicles. What implications does this have for moving to renewable energy for other countries, particularly countries that are slower to take up net zero targets, like Australia? What are the health benefits of electric vehicles? Are there any unintended consequences that should be considered?

Global context: India

India is moving rapidly towards decarbonization with a net zero target for 2070. Some of the most impressive targets have been set by India, compared to other advanced economies. There is an ongoing relationship between Australia and India to develop clean energy and climate technology. For example, for research and construction of turbines, there needs to be security of supply of minerals; Australia is a major supplier of minerals through clean energy supply chains. India has lithium deposits but needs Australia because it has more advanced mineral extraction technology. The largest polluters in both countries are getting clear messages. Yet the relationship is complicated because India still relies on coal and Australia is still exporting large amounts of coal. To move both countries towards net zero targets, more collaboration and policy need to be developed inter and intra both countries to achieve a better, cleaner world.

Let's finish

This chapter has teased out the interconnectedness of housing and energy, drawing on examples from the Global South and Australia. By exploring housing affordability and instability, homelessness and urbanization, energy costs and efficiencies, transitions to renewable energy, and how different demographics are affected by the policies and practices geared towards these issues, this chapter demonstrated how contemporary approaches appealing to individual responsibility and economic rationalities fall short. What is needed is an understanding of collective practices transcending national boundaries that enable just social transformations benefitting all people and communities on a planetary scale.

Summary

In this chapter, you have learnt about the health impacts of housing and energy policies, particularly on people experiencing social disadvantage. Key areas of focus included impacts of urbanization, housing unaffordability and instability, especially taking into account the experiences of Indigenous people and communities, slum dwellers in the Global South and an emergent cohort of people facing the prospect of losing their homes for the first time. We also outlined the health implications of energy policy, transitioning to renewable energy, and the consequences of poor energy infrastructures. The learning objectives for this chapter are summarized here:

- Understand how political factors affect the health of individuals and communities via differential access to appropriate housing and sustainable sources of energy.

The chapter provided examples fleshing out the relations between housing and energy policies, and health outcomes for different people, types of households, and communities.

- Analyse the dynamics between negative health impacts of poor housing and energy infrastructures, and the socio-political landscapes they are embedded in.

The chapter discussed how policy responses are inflected by how problems around housing and energy are framed. Specifically, the chapter highlighted how narratives of individual responsibility and the commodification of public goods underpin policy and practice.

- Assess the logics underpinning housing and energy policy decisions in their repercussions for the health of different demographics within various geopolitical contexts.

The chapter debated contemporary approaches to addressing housing affordability and quality, for example, through fiscal and monetary mechanisms. It also highlighted the tensions arising from narratives emphasizing global community and progress and the rights of urban poor in megacities and gentrified neighbourhoods.

- Critique the economic rationalities informing monetary and fiscal solutions to housing and energy issues from a political determinants of health perspective.

The chapter has laid the foundations for critiquing proposed policy solutions to housing and energy crises that apply economic rationalities, for example, the commodification of public goods and faith in market dynamics, as capable of addressing supply issues.

- Propose alternative conceptual frameworks to address the pressing necessity to meet the energy and housing needs in all communities on a planetary scale.

The chapter encouraged reflections on viable alternatives to pressing issues of housing and energy faced by communities in developing and developed countries alike. The chapter has engaged with conceptualizations that promote a shift from individualized and interventionist approaches towards collective practices and community-led social transformation.

Tutorial exercises

- Working in a small team, discuss the RBA governor's quote above. Identify the underlying logic of the governor's argument. From a political determinants of health perspective, discuss the health repercussions for people living on a low income. What counterargument could you level at the apparent inevitability of exacerbating the housing affordability crisis through monetary political decisions?
- Watch the movie *Nomadland* (Zhao, 2022). In your tutorial, develop a brief summary of instances where housing as a political determinant is shown to have significant health impacts in the movie. How are these dynamics differentiated across demographics, such as gender, age, and ethnicity? Following from the summary and consideration of demographics, discuss if the

main protagonist could be considered homeless. Based on this discussion, suggest key criteria for a contemporary definition of homelessness.
- Divide the tutorial into two groups. Each group will be assigned the task of developing policy levers for energy transformation towards renewables. The key task is to consider the impact on workers who are in fossil fuel industries and their communities. What will the impact on these workers and the community look like? Think in terms of the demographics of these workers and these regions. What are the risks? What support needs to be put in place? What are the politics of ensuring a 'just' transition instead of just another transition?

Acknowledgements

This work was supported by the Australian Research Council through the Centre of Excellence for Children and Families over the Life Course (CE200100025).

Further reading

Bacchi, C. (2009). *Policy analysis: What is the problem represented to be?* Frenchs Forest: Pearson.
Boo, K. (2012). *Behind the beautiful forevers: Life, death, and hope in a Mumbai undercity.* New York: Random House.
Global Forest Watch. (n.d.). Forest monitoring designed for action. Available at: https://www.globalfor estwatch.org/
Parsell, C., Clarke, A., & Kuskoff, E. (2023). Understanding responses to homelessness during COVID-19: An examination of Australia. *Housing Studies*, 38(1), 8–21.
Plage, S., Perrier, R., Bubenik, A., Baker, K., Stambe, R.-M., Kuskoff, E., & Parsell, C. (2023). Health Home Hope: A photographic exhibition on housing and health. West End, Brisbane: The University of Queensland. Available at: https://lifecoursecentre.org.au/news/showcasing-care-at-the-heart-of-hom eless-communities/
Zhao, C. (2020). *Nomadland.* Searchlight Pictures.

References

Anglicare. (2022). *Rental Affordability Snapshot. National Report.* Available at: www.anglicare.asn.au/p ublications/rental
Australian Government. Department of Health and Aged Care. (n.d.). Alcohol throughout life. Available at: https://www.health.gov.au/topics/alcohol/alcohol-throughout-life/alcohol-and-aboriginal-and-torres-strait-islander-peoples
Baker, E., Lester, L., Beer, A., & Bentley, R. (2019). An Australian geography of unhealthy housing. *Geographical Research*, 57(1), 40–51. https://doi.org/10.1111/1745-5871.12326
Chamberlain, C., Marriott, R., & Campbell, S. (2016). Why we need to support Aboriginal women's choice to give birth on Country. *The Conversation*, 15 June.
Goodall, Z., Reynolds, M., Verroja, P., & Stone, W. (2022). 'We've all done the right things': Under cover, older women tell their stories of becoming homeless. *The Conversation*, 18 August.
Guertler, P., & Smith, P. (2018). Cold homes and excess winter deaths: A preventable public health epi-demic that can no longer be tolerated. Briefing Paper. E3G. Available at: www.e3g.org/publications/cold-homes-and-excess
Hanna, L. (2020). Car accidents, drowning, violence: hotter temperatures will mean more deaths from injury. *The Conversation*, 13 January.
Hanmer, G. (2022). Poorly ventilated buildings are allowed under Australia rules – it's time to fix it. *The Conversation*, 6 September.

Hutchens, G., & Whitson, R. (2023). Higher rents will help reduce rental stress by encouraging to 'economise' on housing, RBA governor says. *ABC News*, 31 May.

Langton, M. (1981). Urbanizing Aborigines: The social scientists' great deception. *Social Alternatives*, 2(2), 16–22.

Lutfun Nahar, L. (2021). To whom does the city belong? Obstacles to right to the city for the urban poor in Bangladesh. *Journal of Contemporary Asia*, 51(4), 638–659.

Mapulanga, A. M., & Naito, H. (2019). Effect of deforestation on access to clean drinking water. *PNAS*, 119(17), 8249–8254.

McPhail-Bell, K., Appo, N., Haymes, A., Bond, C., Brough, M., & Fredericks, B. (2018). Deadly Choices empowering Indigenous Australians through social networking sites. *Health Promotion International*, 33(5), 770–780.

NAEH (National Alliance to End Homelessness). (2022). State of homelessness: 2022. Available at: www.endhomelessness.org

Nicoll, F. (2012). Bad habits: Discourses of addiction and the racial politics of intervention. *Griffith Law Review*, 21(1), 164–189.

OECD (Organisation for Economic Co-operation and Development). (2021). HC3–1 Homeless Population. Available at: www.oecd.org/.../HC3-1-Homeless-population.pdf

Padgett, D. K., Henwood, B. F., & Tsemberis, S. J. (2016). *Housing First: Ending homelessness, Transforming systems, and changing lives*. Oxford: Oxford University Press.

Pawson, H., Clarke, A., Parsell, C., & Hartley, C. (2022). Australian Homelessness Monitor 2022. Available at: apo.org.au/.../2022-12/apo-nid321101_0.pdf

Plage, S., & Parsell, C. (2022). Access to health for people experiencing homelessness. *European Journal of Homelessness*, 16(1), 29–52.

Roussos, E. (2023). Dire homelessness situation in the Northern Territory worsening amid 10-year waits for public housing. *ABC News*, 26 March.

Sansom, G., Barlow, C. F., Daniel, L., & Baker, E. (2023). Social housing temperature conditions and tenant priorities. *Australian Journal of Social Issues*, 1–16.

Tucker, J. M., Vittor, A., Rifai, S., & Valle, D. (2017). Does deforestation promote or inhibit malaria transmission in the Amazon? A systematic literature review and critical appraisal of current evidence. *Philosophical Transactions of the Royal Society B*, 372, 20160125.

UN (United Nations). (2021). The Sustainable Development Goals Report 2021. Available at: www.un.org/en/desa/sustainable-development-goals…

4 Education and Employment

Jonathan Hallett

Health inequities flow from patterns of social stratification—that is, from the systematically unequal distribution of power, prestige and resources among groups in society ... People attain different positions in the social hierarchy according, mainly, to their social class, occupational status, educational achievement and income level.

(Solar & Irwin, 2010)

Learning objectives

After studying this chapter, you should be able to:

1   Analyse the influence of political factors on education funding, policy, and teaching practice with implications for public and planetary health.
2   Synthesise historical and current political arguments regarding the curriculum and content taught in Australian schools.
3   Evaluate the correlation between physical and psychosocial workplace conditions and their effects on health and wellbeing.
4   Analyse the role of trade unions and worker advocacy groups in shaping employment conditions and outcomes.
5   Evaluate the effects of globalisation and technological advancements on changes to employment arrangements and intersections with planetary health.

Snapshot

Education and employment are key determinants of health fundamentally shaped by political decisions and policies. Australian universities exemplify their intersection. Decades of under-funding of public higher education and increasing corporatisation of university management and governance left universities vulnerable when COVID-19 hit. Higher education employees are now dealing with the aftermath of the pandemic, which included significant job losses, restructuring, and a shift towards online and outsourced courses. During the lockdowns, 35,000 jobs are estimated to have been lost as universities aimed to maintain profitability in the face of a significant drop in international student revenue. The resulting escalation in job insecurity, burnout, and stress then culminated in widespread industrial action as university workers negotiated with their managements on wages and working conditions. University workers went on strike at institutions across the country to reform the sector to address long-standing industrial issues such as First Nations employment targets, casualisation, unsafe workloads, and wage theft. These efforts were engaged in rebalancing the power differential

DOI: 10.4324/9781003315490-8

between employers and employees and pressuring national policymakers to increase investment in public education and remove barriers to access.

Let's begin

Contemporary schooling as education, and wage labour as employment, are relatively recent concepts that emerged during the Industrial Revolution. Before this, most people were self-employed, worked in small-scale, family-run businesses or were involved in subsistence economies. The growth of large-scale manufacturing and factory production led to the rise of wage labour. People began to work for wages in factories, mines, and mills, rather than for themselves or for small-scale employers. Colonisation expanded this globally, disrupting Indigenous peoples' traditional economies and communities, and enforcing new paradigms that impacted the interconnectedness of work, environment, and cultural practices. Before European colonisation, the Indigenous peoples of Australia had a diverse and sophisticated set of hunting, gathering, and trading practices that formed the basis of their livelihoods.

The development of new industrial technologies led to a shift in the way work was organised in many countries. During the colonial period, the Australian economy was based on agriculture and extractive industries such as forestry, mining, and whaling. This led to a reliance on so-called 'low-skilled' and low-paid jobs and included forced labour from Indigenous peoples on pastoral properties and in other industries. Factories, mines, and mills needed large numbers of workers to operate new machinery, and the division of labour became more specialised. Thus, employment became a central feature of capitalist economies (Spies-Butcher, Paton, & Cahill, 2012). The relationship between employers and employees, and the concept of working for wages, became the norm. Employment became a key aspect of the social contract, as it provided individuals with a means of earning a living and supporting themselves and their families. The designated working hours shaped the way that households organised and spent their time and resulted in a shift where the type of work people performed became central to their identity, income, and social status (Spies-Butcher et al., 2012).

Changing work also brought about the need for a literate workforce. Thus, governments began to invest in public education. In the past, education was accessible only to the wealthy. Early-stage capitalism forced children to work for wages and later established compulsory education (Spies-Butcher et al., 2012). In the early years of Australia's settlement, there were heated disputes between the Church of England, the Presbyterian Church, and the Roman Catholic Church concerning the allocation of responsibility for educating their members (Thompson, Hogan, & Rahimi, 2019). This conflict persisted until the period between 1872 and 1895, when each colony passed free, compulsory, and secular Education Acts. These Acts sought to end most financial support to church schools and instead made primary education the responsibility of the state. Victoria was the first Australian colony and one of the earliest regions globally to provide this education to children with the implementation of the *Education Act of 1872*. In the 1830s, the British government had also established missions in Australia to provide religious instruction and education to Aboriginal people. Many Indigenous children were taken from their families and forced to live in these missions, where they were taught to adopt the ways of white people and forbidden from using their own language as part of the colonisers' belief that they should be assimilated.

This chapter explores the intersection between politics and health and focuses on education and employment as key determinants. We examine how political decisions impact the quality and accessibility of education and employment opportunities, ultimately influencing health outcomes. By recognising the significance of these political determinants, we can work towards creating evidence-based policy solutions to address health inequalities.

The health impacts of the politics of education and education policy

Purpose

Education can impact health in various ways, including providing knowledge and skills for informed health decisions, creating economic opportunities for access to basic needs, improving social networks for support, enhancing mental and emotional wellbeing, and promoting healthy behaviours within school settings. The conceptual framework created by the Commission on Social Determinants of Health (CSDH) (Figure 4.1) highlighted education as a key structural determinant of health inequities along with occupation and income (Solar & Irwin, 2010).

Policy decisions significantly shape education systems, influencing their structure, funding, access, quality, and equity. These decisions often stem from dominant societal beliefs about education's purpose, its structure, and knowledge. Modern schooling generally aims to equip students with a broad knowledge base and skills, preparing them for higher education and employment while fostering critical thinking and problem-solving. There are various philosophies on the purpose of education, including liberal education for personal development, vocational education for practical skills, socialisation for societal integration, and critical pedagogy for social empowerment and change. Each offers distinct pedagogical approaches with varying emphases on student-centred learning, practical experience, or societal issues. Some argue education's primary role in capitalist societies is to produce a compliant workforce, while others assert its purpose is to nurture engaged, active citizens contributing to societal health and progress.

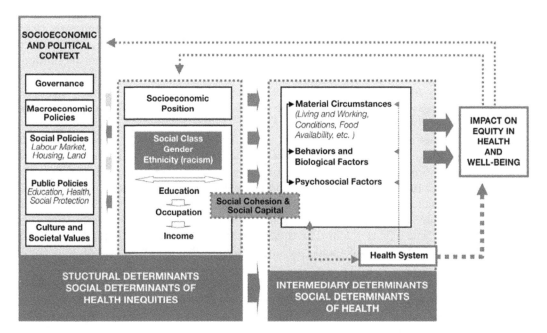

Figure 4.1 Commission on Social Determinants of Health Conceptual Framework
Source: (Solar & Irwin, 2010).

Spotlight: Advocacy action

Saving Northland Secondary College

In 1992, the Victorian Government's budget cuts led to the closure of many schools, including Northland Secondary College, Melbourne's school with the highest Aboriginal population (Knight, 1998). This sparked a campaign to re-open the school, spearheaded by students Muthama Sinnappan and Bruce Foley, community members, legal advisors, and Koori elders, citing indirect racial discrimination. Despite the Equal Opportunity Board ordering the school's re-opening twice, the government appealed each time. During closure, Koori educator Deidre Bux created a volunteer-run 'rebel school' to maintain Koori cultural values and curricula (Knight, 1998). The Rebel School was a volunteer-run example of 'an emancipatory form of culture balanced with the maintenance of basic pedagogical skills in all students' (Knight, 1998, p. 300). After a two-year legal battle that ended in the full Supreme Court (and costing Victorian taxpayers around AUD 4 million), the school re-opened in March 1995.

Pathways

Education pathways are routes that students can take to pursue their educational goals. The Australian education system comprises three sectors: Public, Catholic, and Independent; they all receive government funding (Sinclair & Brooks, 2022). Most Australian students (65.4%) are enrolled in public schools established and managed by state and territory governments through their education departments and authorities, while the remaining third (34.6%) attend private schools run by the Catholic and Independent sectors (Thompson et al., 2019). Australia's high percentage of students enrolled in private schools can be attributed in part to its colonial history and the conflict between the church and state in the late 1800s and early 1900s over the responsibility for educating children, and a series of education policies implemented by the federal government (Thompson et al., 2019). These sectors enrol different proportions and demographics of students. For example, the independent school sector has 14% of all students, with only 6% of these from the lowest quartile of the Socio-Economic Advantage (SEA) index, whereas the public school sector has 66% of students, and 79% come from the lowest quartile of SEA (Sinclair & Brooks, 2022).

School funding is not only about financial inequality but also about social and political factors that impact the distribution of resources at the national, state, and local levels of the education system (Sinclair & Brooks, 2022). In recent decades, there have been considerable increases in federal funding for public and non-government schools; however, increases have been primarily directed towards the latter (Sinclair & Brooks, 2022). This preference for non-government schools was not just an economic decision but also an ideological one. For example, former Prime Minister John Howard stated that he considered the public education system little more than a safety net and guarantor of reasonable quality education (Sinclair & Brooks, 2022).

In many Western countries, education policies have become more utilitarian and focus on vocational education and training (VET) within schools (Down, Smyth, & Robinson, 2019), associating human capital development with economic growth and productivity. Australian schools emphasise competency-based VET to produce 'job-ready' workers (Down et al., 2019). There is a dominant version of vocationalism in Australian schools that focuses on 'VET in Schools' programmes and school-based new apprenticeships (Down et al., 2019). This approach narrows the focus of education and fails to prepare students for a broader range of roles and responsibilities beyond the immediate needs of employers. Down and colleagues argued that this is a deterministic approach of neoliberal ideology that assumes that students must merely adapt to a precarious job market. While schools have a duty to prepare students for the workforce, there is also a moral and political obligation to educate them as responsible and engaged democratic citizens (Down et al., 2019).

Global context: COVID-19 and school closures

The COVID-19 pandemic brought about a staggering disruption to education. The Lancet, Public Health wrote in their (2020) editorial, 'Education: A neglected social determinant of health' that over 80% of students worldwide were impacted by school closures. This exposed significant disparities in the remote learning experience, as the Children's Commissioner for England reported that over half the students were receiving no online lessons and roughly 10% were dedicating less than an hour per day to schoolwork. Beyond formal education, schools are vital spaces for young people's health and wellbeing and foster social and emotional development, physical exercise, safety, and support for those from disadvantaged backgrounds. Prolonged closures have detrimental social and health consequences for children, exacerbate existing inequalities, widen the gap in educational attainment, and reverse progress. The COVID-19 pandemic showed that schools serve purposes beyond providing education and knowledge acquisition. *The Lancet, Public Health* calls on us to re-evaluate the function of schools following the crisis, presenting it as an opportunity to integrate the UN Sustainable Development Goals to achieve 'the interdependent goals of healthy, resilient, and fair societies'.

Attainment

Educational attainment refers to an individual's highest level of completed education, indicating their knowledge, skills, and qualifications. It helps assess career readiness, advancement potential, and social mobility. Higher education levels correlate with lower incidences of chronic and acute illnesses and improved mental and physical health, partly due to the impact of education on career and socioeconomic status. Globally, academic achievement disparity in Australia is more closely tied to students' family and social backgrounds than in many other countries (Sinclair & Brooks, 2022). There are various factors that contribute to lower rates of higher education attainment among, for example, people living in regional and remote areas (Ferguson, 2022). This includes limited local study options for higher education, which forces students to relocate in search of educational opportunities with the associated financial, emotional, and social challenges. Policymakers use education attainment to assess educational systems' efficacy and identify areas for resourcing. The Higher Education Participation and Partnerships Program (HEPPP) was introduced by the Rudd Labor government in 2009 to improve access for low socioeconomic students (LSES) through allocating equity funding to universities, based on the number of LSES enrolled. However, under the Morrison Liberal Government, almost half of HEPPP funding was designated for regional universities, seemingly without distinguishing between affluent and underprivileged rural and regional students (Patty, 2020).

The Australian education system is distinctive in that it is highly privatised in the school and higher education sectors, compared with the systems in other countries. When compared to other OECD countries, Australia's public investment in tertiary education is notably low

(Kniest & Barnes, 2020). OECD data from 2016 reveal that Australia's public investment in tertiary education at 0.75% of GDP is significantly lower than the OECD and European Union averages of approximately 0.93% of GDP, and one of the lowest among all OECD countries. Although the investment in tertiary education in Australia is higher than these averages, it is primarily because of the high proportion of investment from private sources, currently at 65%, which is twice the OECD average of 34%. This is because Australian students pay some of the highest fees in the world to attend public universities.

Higher education policy has experienced significant changes in the last few decades (Kniest & Barnes, 2020). Before the Second World War, state governments were responsible for funding tertiary education. In the 1950s, the Menzies Liberal Government increased funding for universities by providing grants and introducing Commonwealth scholarships. The Whitlam Labor Government took over primary responsibility for funding universities in the 1970s, abolished tuition fees for domestic students, and introduced a Unified National System. In the late 1980s, the Dawkins reforms under Hawke reintroduced tuition fees and income-contingent loans called the Higher Education Contribution Scheme (HECS). Under this framework, universities were allocated a quota of Commonwealth Supported Places (CSPs) to receive a subsidy. A demand-driven system was introduced under the Rudd/Gillard Labor Governments, which allowed universities to enrol as many CSPs as they liked to respond to unmet demand (Kniest & Barnes, 2020). The Abbott/Turnbull Liberal Governments attempted to deregulate university fees and impose funding cuts. Former Education Minister Christopher Pyne's attempts to deregulate university fees were rejected twice by the Senate. Senator Simon Birmingham's 2017 reforms aimed to reduce public funding and increase student contributions but failed to gain parliamentary support. In 2017, the Turnbull Government imposed a funding freeze, which capped government funding for domestic undergraduate students at 2017 levels (Kniest & Barnes, 2020). With the election of the Albanese Labor Government in 2022, higher education policy is on the move again with the initiation of an Australian Universities Accord. This incorporates a broad review of higher education, including a focus on meeting national targets for skills, jobs, and industry-driven research, systemic flaws in VET, insufficient domestic funding, low enrolment rates among certain groups, and the prevalence of casualisation within the academic workforce.

Let's do

Several reforms have been proposed or implemented in higher education policy over the last half-century, including:

1   The Hawke Labor Government's *Higher Education Funding Bill 1988* ended the free tertiary education era initiated by the Whitlam Labor Government in 1974 by introducing the Higher Education Contribution Scheme (HECS), which required domestic students to pay a proportion of the cost of their degrees but defer the payment.
2   The Rudd Labor Government's *Higher Education Support Amendment (Demand-Driven Funding System and Other Measures) Bill 2011* removed government-imposed caps on student places and allowed universities to provide places based on student demand.
3   The Abbott Liberal Government's *Higher Education and Research Reform Amendment Bill 2014* proposed to substantially cut government subsidies for undergraduate study and deregulate course fees to drive competition among universities. This Bill did not pass the Senate.

4   The Morrison Liberal Government introduced the *Higher Education Support Amendment (Job-Ready Graduates and Supporting Regional and Remote Students) Bill 2020* to address skills shortages and support economic recovery following the COVID-19 pandemic.

Select one of these reforms to investigate, and write a brief summary of the reform, including the justification from the government and its impact on universities and students. Discuss the broader implications of these policy changes for the Australian higher education system and contrasting views on the reform.

Attrition

A test of the effectiveness and condition of education and training systems is how many people do not acquire the full range of desired skills and attributes and are left behind. Attrition in the education system takes place when students drop out or withdraw from school before completion of their education. This can occur at any level, from primary to tertiary, and can have significant consequences for the student, their families, and society at large. Attendance levels matter because students who miss a substantial portion of classes are not fully engaged in school. Constantly changing empty desks owing to varying absences also create challenges for teachers who must continually play catch-up. Thus, students get trapped in a vicious cycle of disengagement owing to missed lessons and the lack of involvement because they have fallen behind (Bills & Howard, 2023).

In Australia, school attendance is measured in two ways: attendance rate and level (Bills & Howard, 2023). The former represents the average number of students present at school on any given day, and has consistently declined from 90% in 2014 to 86% in 2022 (Bills & Howard, 2023). The decline becomes more pronounced the farther a school is from a major city, with remote schools experiencing a 10% drop. The latter refers to the percentage of students attending over 90% of the time, which has also been steadily decreasing (Bills & Howard, 2023). In 2014, 8 out of 10 students attended school for over 90% of the time, and in 2022, this number fell to only 5 out of 10 students. This indicates a significant increase in the number of students missing at least a week of school per year. Students may not complete their education for several reasons, including the barriers mentioned above. Young people who have become disinterested or completely disconnected from school (i.e., not attending at all) have expressed feeling out of place in school settings (Bills & Howard, 2023). This sense of not fitting in can be social, academic, or rooted in the perception that the schoolwork they engage in does not align with their future career ambitions. This disconnect between an education experience and the lives of students is not new.

Spotlight: Power dynamics

Safe Schools

The 'Safe Schools' programme, launched in Victoria in 2010, aimed to foster safer environments for lesbian, gay, bisexual, transgender, and intersex (LGBTI) students by offering resources and professional development for educators (Baird & Reynolds, 2021). Initially funded by the Brumby Labor Government and continued by the Baillieu Liberal Government, it was expanded nationally in 2014 by the Abbott Liberal Government through the Safe Schools Coalition Australia (SSCA). However, during the national marriage equality debate in 2016, controversy arose and bipartisan support collapsed (Baird & Reynolds, 2021). Critics called it radical and age-inappropriate, undermining traditional values and parental roles. Supporters argued it was crucial for LGBTI students' wellbeing, countering bullying, and fostering safety. Criticism by an Australian newspaper led to a review. Despite a positive report, the federal government insisted on a requirement for parental consent for student participation. Subsequently, the Victorian government took over funding and federal funding wasn't renewed after 2017 (Baird & Reynolds, 2021).

Successive governments have opted for neoliberal principles instead of social justice as the driving force behind educational reform. Standardisation, measurement, and market choice have become common terms in education, leading to a standardised national curriculum, nationwide testing, and school comparison tools. These reforms have posed challenges for inclusive education, which is expected, given the conflicting values underpinning these different ideological approaches. The National Assessment Program – Literacy and Numeracy (NAPLAN) was introduced by the Rudd/Gillard Labor Government in 2008 and is part of a global trend to increase accountability in education systems (Bills & Howard, 2023). NAPLAN is administered annually to Australian students in Years 3, 5, 7, and 9 by the Australian Curriculum, Assessment and Reporting Authority (ACARA). Mandatory across all school systems, with federal funding dependent on participation, NAPLAN aims to provide an overall indicator of students' literacy and numeracy performance by assessing critical skills for the twenty-first century (Rose et al., 2020).

The 'high-stakes' nature of NAPLAN has resulted in unintended consequences, such as extensive test preparation and covert tactics to exclude or coach students to enhance a school's overall performance (Rose et al., 2020). The publication of results on platforms like *MySchool* fosters national and international competition, which inadvertently narrows down the schools' focus and the types of students they value to be considered 'successful'. This approach limits schools and principals' ability to address the diverse needs, strengths, weaknesses, and interests of individual students and communities (Bills & Howard, 2023). As NAPLAN is tailored for Standard Australian English speakers, it overlooks the linguistic diversity of students proficient in non-standard forms of Australian English, such as 'Kriol' and is deemed linguistically and culturally inappropriate for Indigenous children, especially those in remote communities (Rose et al., 2020). Another issue is the use of a broad LBOTE (Language Background Other Than English) category which is unable to differentiate newly arrived refugee students for targeted funding and assistance (Rose et al., 2020).

The standardised national curriculum has sparked ongoing debates on its content, with critics arguing that it inadequately covers areas such as Western Civilisations, religion, Indigenous history and LGBTI perspectives. While not disputing the criticisms of contemporary schooling that blame the influence of neoliberalism (i.e., individualism, reduced central government responsibility, performativity, competition for funding, evaluation by results), Pirbhai-Illich et al. (2017, p. 13), assert this analysis sidesteps a much longer history; that the 'structures that hold together schools and the academy are colonial and influence what is taught, how it is taught and who does the teaching'. These decisions are made by those in power and result in a curriculum that benefits some but not others and may actively harm public and planetary health. A failure by Federal Liberal governments to prioritise climate change education over the last decade has resulted in no substantive national curriculum on climate change (Gobby & Variyan, 2021). Indeed, under the Federal Education Minister's guidance, references to climate change and embedding sustainability throughout the curriculum were removed from Melbourne Declaration on Educational Goals for Young Australians in 2019 and federal funding and support for school sustainability initiatives and national action plans have also decreased over that time (Gobby & Variyan, 2021).

Indigenous perspective: Education sovereignty

Decolonising education seeks to challenge and reform Eurocentric and colonial perspectives ingrained in education. It aims for inclusivity, integrating Indigenous and non-Western views. Michelle Bishop, a Gamilaroi woman from Western NSW, writes in her (2022) article 'Indigenous education sovereignty: Another way of "doing" education' that while many educational institutions attempt to include Indigenous content in classroom teaching, often in tokenistic ways, there is a lack of professional development to equip teachers to do so thoughtfully and respectfully. Bishop also highlights six core elements describing Indigenous education sovereignty: Pattern Thinking, Country, Time, Relationality, Intergenerational Reciprocity, and Agency. These elements are interconnected and vary according to Place, Peoples, and Knowledge. These components offer a profound comprehension of education sovereignty's potential appearance, thus presenting an alternative approach to education for all learners, rooted in Indigenous belief systems, worldviews, and knowledge frameworks. However, policy approaches like NAPLAN and *MySchool* hinder this needed radical shift, stifling Indigenous language discussions and bi-cultural education, and impacting policies with decolonising potential like Embedding Aboriginal and Torres Strait Islander Perspectives in Schooling (EATSIPS) (Rose et al., 2020).

Let's think

The National School Chaplaincy Program (NSCP) is a government-funded initiative providing pastoral care and support services to improve students' wellbeing in over 3,000 school communities annually. Managed by state and territory governments, the programme has faced public debate since it commenced in 2006 due to its religious nature and concerns about church-state separation. Supporters highlight emotional and spiritual support for disadvantaged students, while critics argue it violates secularism, privileges Christianity, and excludes students from other faiths or those who are not religious. The programme has changed over time, with the Rudd Labor Government incorporating the option of secular Student Welfare Workers in 2010–2011, later removed by the Abbott Liberal Government in 2014. From 2023, under the Albanese Labor Government, the renamed National Student Wellbeing Program (NSWP) again allows hiring Chaplains or secular Student Wellbeing Officers. Reflect on the following: To what extent do the debates surrounding the Australian School Chaplaincy Program reflect a broader tension between the promotion of religious values and the principles of secularism and inclusivity in public education? How can these debates be resolved in a way that supports the wellbeing of students and ensures that public education remains inclusive and accessible to all students, regardless of their religious beliefs and backgrounds?

The health impacts of the politics of employment and employment policy

Structure and regulation

The structure and regulation of employment (exchange of labour for financial remuneration) can have a significant impact on the distribution of wealth, power, and resources, and shape the social and economic relations within a society. Governments have the power to create and enforce legislation, regulations, and policies that can affect employment levels, wages, working conditions, and labour rights. Employment is often the primary source of income for individuals and families, and access to stable and adequate income is a key determinant of health. Work conditions such as hours, demands, and control over one's work environment have a significant impact on people's physical and mental health and lead to health inequalities. Job-related illness is socially created and therefore avoidable; it is possible for employment to be a source of good health and pleasure rather than illness and suffering. It can provide opportunities for social interaction and support networks and generate a sense of purpose and meaning. Ensuring a safe and health-promoting work environment requires identifying the illnesses and injuries related to the workplace and taking action to manage working conditions, set and enforce health and safety standards, and ensure democratic participation in the workplace.

Employment relations exist 'between buyers and sellers of labor as well as the behaviors, outcomes, practices, and institutions that emanate or impinge upon the employment relationship' (Benach et al., 2007, p. 23). These relations operate within historical and political contexts that influence their enactment. Decades of powerful corporate influences and the abandonment of interventionist economic policy and social compacts in favour of neoliberalism by many governments have set up microeconomic rationality as the validating criterion for all aspects of social life (Benach et al., 2007). From the belief that competitive markets produce the best results, neoliberal policies and practices include rejecting public spending as a means to manage unemployment rates. The history of workplace health must be understood in light of this ideology as it sets the terms of debate around workers, work, and the wider economic and social values that influence how we value different forms of labour. Benach et al. (2007, p. 23) suggested that much of this history

> has been characterized by unequal power and conflict between labor and capital [employers, or buyers of labour], the former often represented by unions demanding higher wages, shorter hours, and better working conditions with strikes, and the latter resisting those demands through firings, lockouts, or court injunctions.

A trade union (or labour/workers' union) represents the collective interests of workers in a particular industry or profession. They comprise workers who have banded together to negotiate better wages, benefits (e.g., paid leave, employer contributions to superannuation), and working conditions for their members. Trade unions represent members in negotiations with employers on wages and working conditions (i.e., collective bargaining) and in workplace disputes. Unions have pushed for legislation and policies that benefit workers and the wider community, such as health and safety regulations, minimum wage laws, and universal health care.

The following framework outlines the context for employment relations and its connections to health inequalities (Figure 4.2). It incorporates power relations within and between markets, corporations, governments, and civil society and their influence on the labour market and welfare state. It describes the influence of key political actors and institutions that interact and distribute power and economic resources exclusively to some groups in society through policy decisions that determine the experience that different groups have within the labour market, their access to social protection, and the reality of their work and life conditions. The distribution of resources affects social stratification, opportunities for healthy living, exposure to risks that may cause death, disease, illness, or injury, and access to health care experienced by various social groups (Benach et al., 2007). For example, women encounter unique circumstances and structural obstacles that differ from those faced by men in terms of labour market

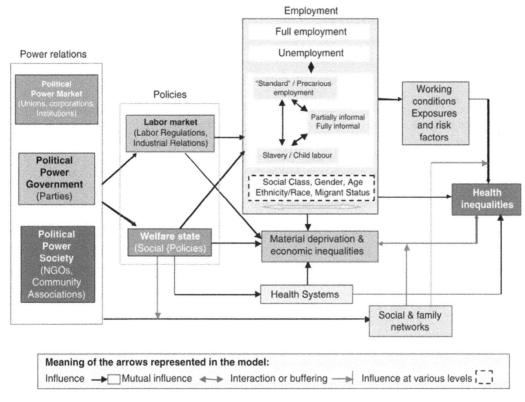

Figure 4.2 Macro-theoretical framework of employment relations and health inequalities
Source: Benach et al. (2007).

participation. Tax and labour market data indicate a significant disparity in the representation of women and men across the workforce, with women being predominantly concentrated in low-paying industries and occupations and insecure employment.

Benach et al. (2007) described the first level of the framework as referring to the different powers that influence the labour market and its characteristics (industrial and labour laws and regulations, collective bargaining, and trade union power), and the welfare state's level of development (the extent to which the state redistributes power through social policies). The key characteristic of Australia's liberal welfare state is that its primary institution is the market (Raphael, 2015). In such a welfare state, fewer economic and social benefits are provided by the government, and universal benefits are scarce, with the government only providing modest benefits to those who are least well-off. As the market is not highly regulated by laws and regulations, the distribution of wages and benefits is more unequal. Another notable characteristic is a comparatively weak labour sector, which is a consequence of the political system enabling the business and corporate sector to hold more economic power than the government (Raphael, 2015). Both institutions are crucial to understanding employment relations as employee wellbeing depends on the labour market and social protection measures available when involuntary unemployment occurs. This framework details how different forms of employment (including full employment, unemployment, precarious employment, and slavery) interact with factors such as social class, gender, age, ethnicity, and migrant status to influence economic inequalities and expose workers to hazardous working conditions.

Spotlight: Other determinants

Gender pay gap

The ongoing pay disparity between men and women in Australia significantly contributes to women's financial disadvantage. The Australia Institute's Centre for Future Work published a recent report, *The Times They Aren't A-Changin* (Littleton & Jericho, 2023), which highlights a 13.3% gender pay gap based on 2022 data. The *Workplace Gender Equality Act 2012* mandates Australian non-public sector organisations with over 100 employees to report yearly on gender equity and remuneration. Recent 2023 reforms included federal public sector organisations. Some local governments, like Sydney, Yarra, Wollongong, and Vincent, are voluntarily improving pay equity and transparency. Reducing the gender pay gap yields economic benefits such as increased productivity, organisational performance, talent retention, improved work environment, and enhanced reputation. Bearing this in mind, research your local government and identify if they voluntarily report gender equity indices in their annual report. Locate the contact details of your local elected council members and write to them with a request to investigate their workforce profile and report publicly on their workforce by employment status and gender, their gender pay gap, and the proportion of women at the management/executive levels. Review the replies you receive with fellow students and discuss any objections.

Occupation

People's occupations exacerbate the risk of poor health. The location, type, and context of their employment have direct impacts on health, which are not evenly distributed across different occupations or social groups. Approximately 200 Australian workers are fatally injured while working each year; in 2021, over 130,000 claims for work-related injury or illness were approved (Safe Work Australia, 2023). Most serious workers' compensation claims occurred in the agriculture, construction, road transport, manufacturing, health care and social assistance, and public administration and safety industries (Safe Work Australia, 2023). Workplaces may expose workers to adverse physical or psychosocial conditions, poor pay or insufficient (or too many) hours, job insecurity, and low job satisfaction (UCL Institute of Health Equity, 2015). Physical risks include physically demanding or dangerous work, repetitive injury, exposure to chemicals and other hazards, long or irregular hours and shift work. For example, contact dermatitis is the most common kind of skin illness caused through occupational exposure to irritants or allergens. Occupational diseases believed to have been eradicated, such as black lung and silicosis, have also re-emerged in Australia. About 7% of Australian workers are at risk of inhaling silica dust (produced through cutting or drilling material such as concrete and pavers), most commonly in mining and the construction industries (Fritschi & Carey, 2022). Manufacturing artificial stone for consumer products like kitchen benchtops is a key source of this risk. Fritschi and Carey (2022) suggested that a specific ban on artificial stone alone can prevent almost 1000 silicosis and 100 lung cancer cases in a single year. Parts of Australia have extreme heat conditions and a changing climate is exacerbating this. Exposure to heat and solar ultraviolet radiation (UVR) are recurring high-risk activities. As many as 1.2 million Australian outdoor workers have up to 10 times the level of exposure to the UVR of indoor workers, which results in 200 melanomas and 34,000 non-melanomas each year (Cancer Council, n.d.).

Long working hours (over 48 hours per week) increases exhaustion, the potential for incidents, and injuries and may impact workers' mental health through stress and depression (UCL Institute of Health Equity, 2015). Fly-in fly-out patterns of work are common in mining industries and the resulting mental health impact compounds with other physical occupational risks. Shift work is common among many occupations and has well-established negative impacts on health, including reduced mental health, increased fatigue, lower sleep quality and quantity, and increased cardiovascular disease risk (UCL Institute of Health Equity, 2015). The process of increasing the quantity, intensity, or pace of work, resulting in an increased workload and greater demands on workers is called work intensification and can lead to higher levels of stress, burnout, and job dissatisfaction, and physical and psychological health problems. The rise in hybrid and remote work fuelled by COVID-19 has increased the challenges in managing workplace hazards beyond the traditional workplace controlled by the employer.

Psychosocial stress at work can result from workplace conflict, bullying, harassment, discriminatory practices, restricted participation in decision-making, and the lack of autonomy. These appear to occur most frequently in occupations in public administration and safety, and health care and social assistance (Safe Work Australia, 2023). Many workplaces are rigidly hierarchical, which has resulted in many workers having little control over their work. This has been shown to have a social gradient where low socioeconomic status is linked to less control at work, which is associated with declines in physical functioning and increases in absences owing to illness, mental illness, cardiovascular disease, and metabolic syndrome. Being underpaid and having low control in a demanding job increase chronic stress responses and negative emotions, which can have long-term health consequences (UCL Institute of Health Equity, 2015). Higher levels of job satisfaction lead to increased productivity and creativity and a reduction in absenteeism (UCL Institute of Health Equity, 2015). Having a low income has obvious implications for poor health. This may be through a reduced capacity to afford quality housing, food, and health care as well as the effects of stress resulting from an inadequate income. There may be a feedback loop where poor health causes lower income (UCL Institute of Health Equity, 2015). Additional stress can be caused through precarious employment or the lack of job security. Those with job uncertainty or precarity report poorer health than those with secure employment (UCL Institute of Health Equity, 2015).

Spotlight: Other determinants

Welfare and poverty

Australia's welfare system offers conditional means-tested support to disadvantaged groups through mechanisms like Newstart Allowance, Youth Allowance and the Pension. Although Australia's welfare costs are lower than many other nations, poverty is prevalent among those reliant on welfare. Poverty, a lack of basic necessities for a minimum standard of living, can be measured through income, consumption, or social exclusion. The Henderson Poverty Line is a standard measure in Australia with different set income levels for different types of households (Melbourne Institute, 2022). Apart from pensioners, current maximum welfare benefits don't raise recipients above the poverty line, which poses barriers to accessing employment.

Employment

Employment trends reflect and deepen the socioeconomic divide. There are significant inequalities in access to opportunities in the labour market. Those with higher incomes have more disposable income, whereas those with lower incomes allocate a greater proportion of their income to necessities. The differences in the standard of living result in inequalities in health, owing to the impact on the access to and affordability of necessities, such as housing, food, and health care. The unemployment rate is calculated as the percentage of people in a particular location who are of working age, but do not currently have a job and are actively looking for one. This definition can vary and may not include individuals with long-term illnesses who could work given appropriate working conditions, parents who could work if childcare was accessible, or those who want to work, but face barriers finding work. Being employed for just one hour disqualifies an individual from this statistic, regardless of the need for additional hours (Hail, 2021). Unemployment statistics are criticised for not reflecting the true extent of the problem or for their unqualified use as an indicator and need to be supplemented with other concepts like under-employment (Hail, 2021). Underemployment is a condition of individuals who are working (therefore counted as employed) but not in jobs that fully utilise their skills, qualifications, and experience or those who want (and are available) to work additional hours. Over 30% of the Australian workforce is in part-time employment and underemployment has consistently exceeded unemployment for nearly 20 years (Hail, 2021).

Therefore, a better measure of employment policy success (or failure) is said to be the underutilisation rate (unemployment and underemployment combined) (Hail, 2021). The underutilisation rate in Australia has been below 10% only twice briefly since 1982, meaning for 40 years, job creation has been insufficient to meet the needs of job seekers (Hail, 2021). Hail argues that, despite a large number of people searching for non-existent jobs and many in insecure employment, politicians from both major parties have praised their job creation schemes, sometimes even claiming full employment. Rather than addressing successive governments' failure to ensure job availability, politicians have allowed unemployment to persist while implementing and maintaining a punitive approach towards the unemployed, blaming their motivation (Hail, 2021).

Rising disparities in Australian employment amplify socioeconomic gaps in income and wealth. Unemployment rates are highest among those of older age, those with disability and/or poor mental health, Aboriginal and Torres Strait Islander people, and single parents. After a period of unemployment, someone is more likely to have insecure work in the future. These groups are at a higher risk of being employed in low-paid, low-quality jobs that offer few prospects for growth and involve labour in hazardous conditions. People who lose their jobs have significant income drops that last even after they find new employment. Five years after a three-month period of unemployment, workers with solid job histories will still have an 11% reduced labour income, and over five years, the cumulative effect is comparable to over a year's worth of lost wages (Coates & Ballantyne, 2022). Unemployment's population-level impact compounds as decreased consumer spending can cause additional job losses. Workforce participation programmes, such as Work for the Dole, cannot address this alone, as many welfare recipients (e.g., single parents, persons with disabilities, long-term jobless, those with criminal records) encounter barriers to finding suitable or sufficient work. Insufficient welfare payments add financial stress to the disadvantaged during their search for employment.

Let's think

The Raise the Rate for Good campaign (https://raisetherate.org.au/), led by the Australian Council of Social Service with broad support, aims to raise the Job Seeker Payment. A recent Senate enquiry also endorsed a raise to alleviate poverty. The increase would boost the economy via spending and job growth. However, there is significant opposition from some government officials and business groups, who argue that increasing unemployment benefits would disincentivise people from seeking work and lead to a rise in welfare dependency. In 2022, the Albanese Labor Government agreed to establish an Economic Inclusion Advisory Panel to review unemployment benefits and advise on economic inclusion challenges before each budget. As a Panel member, evaluate the evidence and advise on potential unemployment benefit increases. Consider factors such as cost of living, employment rates, and the potential socio-economic impacts of an increase.

Before the COVID-19 recession, Australia's economy was sluggish with low inflation, high underemployment and unemployment and stagnant wage rises. However, compared to prior recessions, Australia recovered far more quickly. By early 2022, the unemployment rate was barely 4%, which was close to a 50-year low (Coates & Ballantyne, 2022). Low unemployment brings greater bargaining power for workers as there is not a large pool of unemployed people willing to work for lower wages or poorer conditions. The different ways in which labour/ capital relations may be negotiated is called collective bargaining. The level of wage-setting – that is, whether wages are decided at the personal, individual workplace, industry, or whole private sector level – is crucial in explaining pay disparity (Benach et al., 2007). Additional factors include the density of union membership and percentage of the workforce covered by collective bargaining agreements.

In countries with high union membership, strong unions lead to better social protection for workers, more supportive government labour policies, and greater job security. For instance, the two-thirds difference in the increase in pay disparity between the US and Canada is because of the far more severe decrease in unionisation in the former (Benach et al., 2007). In Australia, despite trade union membership falling from 41% in 1992 to 12.5% in 2022, employees who were union members in their primary job earned a median weekly income of AUD 1,520 when compared to AUD 1,208 earned by those who were not (Australian Bureau of Statistics, 2022). However, according to Stanford (2018) union members in Australia face substantial legal, administrative, and economic obstacles in conducting industrial action as part of collective bargaining (among the harshest in any industrialised nation). Industrial action refers to collective actions taken by employees, such as strikes, work stoppages, and slowdowns, as a form of protest or bargaining tool in negotiations in response to issues concerning their employment, such as wages, hours, and working conditions.

Indigenous perspective: The Wave Hill Walk-Off

The Wave Hill Walk-Off (1966–1973), led by Indigenous Gurindji stockmen, including elder Vincent Lingiari, against Vestey's British pastoral company in Australia, was a landmark in Indigenous rights. Protesting poor wages, working conditions, and land theft, strikers were supported by trade unions and activists. They demanded their land back, camped at sacred site Daguragu, and attracted global attention. In 1975, the Australian government, under Gough Whitlam, returned part of Wave Hill Station to the Gurindji, a pivotal moment in Indigenous land rights. The strike also improved Indigenous workers' conditions in the pastoral industry and marked a significant moment in the Australian labour movement's history. Watch the Living Black episode on the Wave Hill Walk Off: https://www.youtube.com/watch?v= FEDFN-LKY10

Decisions made by governments to limit or ban industrial conflicts have reduced the occurrence of organised industrial action in Australia. In proportion to the population, the number of work stoppages has declined by 97% since the 1970s (Stanford, 2018). Industrial action is regulated in Australia by the *Fair Work Act 2009* and is subject to a range of legal restrictions. Without the ability to reinforce their demands with a credible threat of collective action, unions' power to secure improved wages and working conditions from employers is significantly weakened (Stanford, 2018). Although work stoppages may sometimes be disruptive or expensive, Stanford argued that they are an inherent aspect of a free collective bargaining system in which workers can withhold their labour together to counteract the power of employers. In the post-war economic boom period when strikes were more frequent, the cost of disputes was balanced by the benefits of rising wages through collective bargaining. However, the current focus of the Fair Work Commission on minimising the economic impact of potential industrial disputes appears to overlook the broader costs of wage stagnation and inequality in the labour market (Stanford, 2018).

The gig economy

The gig economy has grown during a period of economic uncertainty, with many workers seeking more flexible and autonomous forms of work to supplement their income or replace lost jobs. Gig work involves a worker undertaking tasks (e.g., food delivery or ride share) through digital platforms that connect them with businesses seeking completion of specific jobs (Murphy, 2022). These platforms take a share of the earnings, control the platform's brand, and manage the worker-client relationship (e.g., through rating systems and non-circumvention clauses). This distinguishes gig work from freelance work or conventional independent contracting, as gig workers do not develop or manage their own reputations or businesses (Murphy, 2022). As they are typically classified as self-employed contractors rather than employees of the platform/companies, gig workers are usually ineligible to receive benefits meant for employees. The Australian Greens have argued that the Fair Work Commission should be given the authority to apply minimum wages, benefits, and conditions to contractors, ensuring that workers receive equal remuneration and conditions regardless of their employee classification status (Murphy, 2022).

Gig work is just one type of precarious employment, which includes any form of employment that lacks a permanent contract, including those with fixed-term or temporary contracts, whether full- or part-time. Kreshpaj et al. (2020) have identified key characteristics of precarious employment encompassing various disadvantages in different forms of employment, including job insecurity (e.g., temporary, multiple jobs), inadequate income (e.g., low pay, fluctuations in earnings), and limited rights and protections (e.g., lack of union representation and absence of benefits). With the decline in trade unions and erosion of labour protections, precarious employment has been on the rise in many countries in recent decades and can have negative impacts on workers' physical and mental health, financial stability, and overall wellbeing. The composition of skills in the Australian labour market has undergone a transformation in recent decades, with a notable decline in manufacturing jobs, and an increase in industries such as retail trade, hospitality, health care, and social services, which also have a higher likelihood of offering casual jobs. Nonetheless, the climate crisis and the urgent need to transition to renewable technologies present numerous opportunities to reshape industries and employment conditions.

Global context: Just transition

The McGowan/Cook Labor Government in Western Australia is transitioning Collie from coal-dependency to new industries, guided by a just transition framework. As coal plants phase out by 2029, the Collie Transition Package, including an Industrial Transition Fund, aims to attract industries and generate jobs, with additional support for local training via the expanded Collie Jobs and Skills Centre. The just transition concept, originated by labour unions and environmental justice groups, promotes phasing out harmful industries while providing fair job alternatives (Mascarenhas-Swan, 2017). The Just Transition Alliance in the US pioneered discussions between workers in polluting industries and affected communities in the 1990s. A just transition transforms the economy to foster ecological restoration, community resilience, and social equity (Mascarenhas-Swan, 2017).

Let's finish

Public health professionals play a crucial leadership role in responding to the impacts of climate change and the more recent COVID-19 disruptions. These challenges have worsened global health and education disparities, hindering progress towards the United Nations 2030 Sustainable Development Goals. The future of our education systems and working lives is inextricably connected to how we respond to climate change and global inequities in health. Bridging health and wellbeing gaps between Indigenous and non-Indigenous communities remains a top priority in Australasia and Indigenous education sovereignty is essential for cultural survival and celebration.

Investing in higher education ensures future prosperity across economic, social, and cultural dimensions. Such investments benefit individuals, businesses, governments, regions, and society, leading to higher earnings, a productive workforce, business opportunities, and regional employment. Governments gain increased tax revenue, while society enjoys economic advantages such as export income, growth, and lower unemployment rates. The social benefits include better health, lower crime rates, international connections, and increased civic participation. Education can be transformed into a tool to empower the working class, foster critical thinking, and promote collective action against oppressive systems. Embracing a climate-resilient economy will not only protect our planet, but also provide opportunities for job growth and innovation. Economic transformation requires reducing emissions, transitioning industries to clean energy, and protecting homes and infrastructure from climate-related disasters. However, most people are trapped in a labour market that prioritises corporate profits over urgent societal and environmental needs, while real wages fall. A punitive unemployment system perpetuates this cycle by keeping workers in poverty and desperation rather than providing adequate assistance. To address the climate crisis and foster a more equitable society, we must focus on implementing solutions that challenge the status quo and prioritise the wellbeing of people and the planet.

Summary

The complex interplay between politics, education, and employment significantly influences human and planetary health. Government policies and funding decisions, influenced by ideology, economic priorities, and social values, determine education's accessibility, quality, outcomes, and opportunities, impacting health. Similarly, political ideologies shape employment via policies on labour market regulation, minimum wage, social security, and taxation, affecting job availability, security, conditions, and remuneration. These aspects impact workers' health through stress levels, occupational hazard exposure, and access to safety resources. Low income, job insecurity, and lack of workplace control lead to poor health outcomes. Rising employment disparities in Australia magnify income and wealth inequalities across socio-economic groups. Workforce programmes alone cannot resolve this issue, and insufficient welfare payments exacerbate difficulties for disadvantaged individuals.

Having read this chapter, you should now be able to:

- Analyse the influence of political factors on education funding, policy and teaching practice with implications for public and planetary health.
- Synthesise historical and current political arguments regarding the curriculum and content taught in Australian schools.
- Evaluate the correlation between physical and psychosocial workplace conditions and their effects on health and wellbeing.
- Analyse the role of trade unions and worker advocacy groups in shaping employment conditions and outcomes.
- Evaluate the effects of globalisation and technological advances on changes to employment arrangements and intersections with planetary health.

Further reading

Australian Council of Social Service (ACOSS) and UNSW Sydney. Research and insights into poverty & inequality in Australia. Available at: https://povertyandinequality.acoss.org.au/

Australian Council of Trade Unions (ACTU). Available at: https://www.actu.org.au/.

Bishop, M. (2022). Indigenous education sovereignty: Another way of 'doing' education. *Critical Studies in Education*, 63(1), 131–146.

Connell, R. (2022). Remaking universities: Notes from the sidelines of catastrophe. *The Conversation*. Available at: http://theconversation.com/remaking-universities-notes-from-the-sidelines-of-catastrophe-175920

Crawford, G., Hallett, J., Price, T., Hannelly, T., & Pollard, C. (2022). Advocacy and the workforce. In P. Liamputtong (ed.), *Public health: Local and global perspectives*. Cambridge: Cambridge University Press.

Gerrard, J., & Threadgold, S. (2022). The concept of class is often avoided in public debate, but it's essential for understanding inequality. *The Conversation*. Available at: http://theconversation.com/the-concept-of-class-is-often-avoided-in-public-debate-but-its-essential-for-understanding-inequality-187777

International Labour Organization. (2023). World employment and social outlook: Trends 2023. Available at: http://www.ilo.org/global/research/global-reports/weso/WCMS_865332/lang–en/index.htm

Littleton, E., & Jericho, G. (2023). *The Times They Aren't A-Changin*. Manuca, ACT: Centre for Future Work, The Australia Institute.

Long, S. (2017). Have right to strike laws gone too far? *ABC News*, 20 March. Available at: https://www.abc.net.au/news/2017-03-21/have-the-right-to-strike-laws-gone-too-far/8370980

Taylor, J., Roiko, A., Coombe, L., Oldroyd, J., Hallett, J., Murray, Z., Nona, F., Canuto, C., Amato Ali, D., Crawford, G., & Gurnett, T. (2023). Council of Academic Public Health Institutions Australasia: Public health education for a sustainable future 'Call to Action', 2021. *Australian and New Zealand Journal of Public Health*, 47(2), 10042.

References

Australian Bureau of Statistics. (2022). Trade union membership. Available at: https://www.abs.gov.au/statistics/labour/earnings-and-working-conditions/trade-union-membership/latest-release (accessed 15 December 2022).

Baird, B., & Reynolds, R. (2021). Unsafe subjects: The constitution of young LGBTQ political subjects in the Safe School controversy. *Australian Historical Studies*, 52(3), 402–419.

Benach, J., Muntaner, C., & Santana, V. (2007). Employment conditions and health inequalities: Final report to the WHO Commission on Social Determinants of Health (CSDH). Employment Conditions Knowledge Network (EMCONET).

Bills, A., & Howard, N. (2023). School attendance rates are dropping. We need to ask students why. *The Conversation*, 26 February. Available at: http://theconversation.com/school-attendance-rates-are-dropp ing-we-need-to-ask-students-why-200537

Cancer Council. (n.d.). UV radiation at work. Available at: https://www.cancer.org.au/cancer-informa tion/causes-and-prevention/workplace-cancer/uv-radiation-at-work (accessed 15 December 2022).

Coates, B., & Ballantyne, A. (2022). No one left behind: Why Australia should lock in full employmen *t*. Grattan Institute. Available at: https://grattan.edu.au/report/no-one-left-behind-why-australia-shoul d-lock-in-full-employment/

Down, B., Smyth, J., & Robinson, J. (2019). Problematising vocational education and training in schools: Using student narratives to interrupt neoliberal ideology. *Critical Studies in Education*, 60(4), 443–461.

Ferguson, H. (2022). Regional and remote higher education: A quick guide (Research Paper Series, 2021– 2022). Parliamentary Library, Australian Government. Available at: https://parlinfo.aph.gov.au/pa rlInfo/download/library/prspub/8543739/upload_binary/8543739.pdf;fileType=application%2Fpdf#sea rch=%22Education%22

Fritschi, L., & Carey, R. (2022). Banning artificial stone could prevent 100 lung cancers and 1,000 cases of silicosis, where dust scars the lungs. *The Conversation*. Available at: http://theconversation.com/ba nning-artificial-stone-could-prevent-100-lung-cancers-and-1-000-cases-of-silicosis-where-dust-sca rs-the-lungs-182420

Gobby, B., & Variyan, G. (2021). Curriculum is a climate change battleground and states must step in to prepare students. *The Conversation*, 24 November.Available at: http://theconversation.com/curriculum -is-a-climate-change-battleground-and-states-must-step-in-to-prepare-students-172392

Hail, S. (2021). The return of full employment. *Australian Fabians*, 2. Available at: https://www.fabians. org.au/afr2_steven_hail

Kniest, P., & Barnes, A. (2020). National Tertiary Education Union (NTEU) 2020–21 Pre-Budget Submission. National Tertiary Education Union. Available at: https://treasury.gov.au/2020-21-pre-budget-submissions

Knight, T. (1998). Public knowledge: Public education: Northland Secondary College versus the State. *International Journal of Inclusive Education*, 2(4), 295–308.

Kreshpaj, B., Orellana, C., Burström, B., Davis, L., Hemmingsson, T., Johansson, G., Kjellberg, K., Jonsson, J., Wegman, D. H., & Bodin, T. (2020). What is precarious employment? A systematic review of definitions and operationalizations from quantitative and qualitative studies. *Scandinavian Journal of Work, Environment & Health*, 46(3), 235–247.

Littleton, E., & Jericho, G. (2023). *The Times They Aren't A-Changin*. Manuca, ACT: Centre for Future Work, The Australia Institute.

Mascarenhas-Swan, M. (2017). The case for a just transition. In D. Fairchild, & A. Weinrub (eds), *Energy democracy: Advancing equity in clean energy solutions*. Washington, DC: Island Press/Center for Resource Economics, pp. 37–56. https://doi.org/10.5822/978-1-61091-852-7_3

Melbourne Institute. (2022). Poverty lines: Australia (June Quarter 2022). Melbourne: The University of Melbourne.

Murphy, J. (2022). Regulating the 'gig' economy as a form of employment (Australia). Parliamentary Library, Australian Government. Available at: https://www.aph.gov.au/About_Parliament/Parliamenta ry_departments/Parliamentary_Library/pubs/BriefingBook47p/GigEconomy

Patty, A. (2020). Western Sydney students to lose millions of dollars from university funding reforms. *The Sydney Morning Herald*, 28 September. Available at: https://www.smh.com.au/business/workplace/wes tern-sydney-students-to-lose-millions-of-dollars-from-university-funding-reforms-20200923-p55ydt.html

Pirbhai-Illich, F., Pete, S., & Martin, F. (2017). Culturally responsive pedagogies: Decolonization, indigeneity and interculturalism. In F. Pirbhai-Illich, S. Pete, & F. Martin (eds), *Culturally responsive pedagogy: Working towards decolonization, indigeneity and interculturalism*New York: Springer International Publishing, pp. 3–25.

Raphael, D. (2015). The political economy of health: A research agenda for addressing health inequalities in Canada. *Canadian Public Policy*, 41(Supplement 2), S17–S25.

Rose, J., Low-Choy, S., Singh, P., & Vasco, D. (2020). NAPLAN discourses: A systematic review after the first decade. *Discourse: Studies in the Cultural Politics of Education*, 41(6), 871–886.

Safe Work Australia. (2023). Australian Work Health and Safety (WHS) Strategy 2023–2033. Canberra: Australian Government. Available at: https://www.safeworkaustralia.gov.au/sites/default/files/2023-02/Australian%20WHS%20Strategy%202023-33.pdf

Sinclair, M. P., & Brooks, J. S. (2022). School funding in Australia: A critical policy analysis of school sector influence in the processes of policy production. *Education Policy Analysis Archives*, 30, 16.

Solar, O., & Irwin, A. (2010). A conceptual framework for action on the social determinants of health. Social Determinants of Health Discussion Paper 2 (Policy and Practice). Geneva: World Health Organization. Available at: https://apps.who.int/iris/handle/10665/44489

Spies-Butcher, B., Paton, J., & Cahill, D. (2012). *Market society: Theory, history, practice.* Cambridge: Cambridge University Press.

Stanford, J. (2018). Historical data on the decline in Australian industrial disputes. Manuca, ACT: Centre for Future Work, The Australia Institute. Available at: https://australiainstitute.org.au/report/historical-data-on-the-decline-in-australian-industrial-disputes/

The Lancet. Public Health (2020). Education: A neglected social determinant of health. *The Lancet. Public Health*, 5(7), e361.

Thompson, G., Hogan, A., & Rahimi, M. (2019). Private funding in Australian public schools: A problem of equity. *The Australian Educational Researcher*, 46(5), 893–910.

UCL Institute of Health Equity. (2015). *Local action on health inequalities: Promoting good quality jobs to reduce health inequalities.* London: Public Health England.

5 Media and Misinformation

Melissa Sweet and Megan Williams

> Imagine a global communication network that was monitored with care and empathy as opposed to hate, violence and controversy.
>
> (Bronwyn Carlson, 2022)

Learning objectives

After studying this chapter, you should be able to:

1 Understand the distinctive features of the Australian media ecosystem and the global context.
2 Critique the media landscape, including historical, corporate, cultural and systemic ideologies.
3 Analyse the impacts of misinformation and disinformation on planetary health.
4 Critically synthesise how public health can contribute to a healthier media landscape.

Snapshot

The media, a term encompassing traditional news media as well as social media, is an influential determinant of public and planetary health, including through its impacts upon community knowledge and participation, and political and policy processes and outcomes. It is also a powerful force in creating and disseminating misinformation. The historic and ongoing legacy of colonisation shapes the nature of the media landscape in Australia, with adverse outcomes for the health and wellbeing of people, communities, democracy, and the environmental determinants of health. This chapter consciously uses decolonising methodologies to examine media and misinformation. Decolonising methodologies are an appropriate and useful framework for examining the political determinants of planetary health generally, and specifically in relation to the media and misinformation, with the aim of encouraging transformative change (Sweet, 2017).

Decolonising methodologies respect the rights of Indigenous people and acknowledge their highly developed techniques for intergenerational knowledge transfer and holistic caring for Country, which is essential for planetary health. Elements of decolonising methodologies include privileging the voices and knowledges of Indigenous peoples, a commitment to self-determination, caring for Country and other cultural determinants of health, cultural safety and anti-racism. Other elements include reflexivity, and trauma-informed and strengths-based approaches (Sweet, 2017). The plural term, 'decolonising methodologies', recognises that there is no single pathway involved, as every journey will be different, depending upon starting

DOI: 10.4324/9781003315490-9

points and positioning. Decolonising methodologies require authors and users of information to understand their own standpoint from which others' perspectives are interpreted, and to use local Indigenous peoples' cultural protocols.

We therefore begin this chapter with an Acknowledgement of Country; it has been written on the unceded sovereign lands of the Wiradjuri peoples, the Gadigal people of the Eora nation, the Bediagal people of the Dharug nation, the Melukerdee people of lutruwita and the Ngadjuri people. We belong to Croakey Health Media, with Melissa the Editor-in-Chief and Megan a contributing editor and Board Chair. Meg is Wiradjuri through paternal family, with English and Irish heritage, and is a trained social scientist and professor of Indigenous Health. Melissa is a public health journalist of English, Scottish and Chinese ancestry, and her family, ancestors and profession of journalism have contributed to the ongoing legacy of colonisation. Melissa seeks to incorporate decolonising methodologies into her life and work, including through journalism practice and research.

Let's begin

In this chapter we examine how a toxic news and information ecosystem is influenced by the dominance of corporate and colonial interests that shape the political determinants of planetary health. We investigate the implications for planetary health of power imbalances in the news and information ecosystem, and also analyse the growing problems of misinformation and disinformation in the context of both of the dominant market power of Big Tech and as longstanding strategies of colonisation. In doing so, we focus on caring for Country as the foundation for planetary health, acknowledging that the latter is a relatively recent concept. Caring for Country is an holistic concept integrating knowledges that have evolved over millennia, and that encompasses understanding and respect for interconnections between all beings and land, water, air and a spirituality and meanings for identity and the cultural determinants of health.

A focus on caring for Country is in keeping with decolonising methodologies and a growing global appreciation of the importance of centring Indigenous knowledges and ways of knowing, being and doing in addressing the planetary health crisis. Institutions and organisations across sectors, including health and the media, are moving to more systematically embed Indigenous knowledges in curriculum, frameworks, research, workforce design, policy, and models of practice. Aboriginal and Torres Strait Islander Elders ask that 'no matter where we come from, we seek to deepen our connection to each other and the Country that nourishes us' (Pascoe & Shukuroglou, 2020, p. ix). But it is obvious from the previous two centuries in Australia that neither the privileging of individuals' relationship with Country, nor the centring and loving of Country itself have occurred. It is not a norm or a reality that mainstream media companies provide the time or resources for the types of 'rich conversations, long walks, humour and vulnerability' (Pascoe & Shukuroglou, 2020, p. ix) that Country can inspire in human communications. The sheer absence of communications about connections between Country, public health and the role of the media is clear. Country has been rendered invisible and its fundamental roles in human wellbeing overlooked. Knowledges about the role of Country in producing humans' identities, languages, spirituality and health are all but gone from public access. Even social media platforms, promoted for connecting people, often undermine humans' own need for connection in ways that are damaging for individual, public and planetary health (Williams & Sweet, 2021).

On the other hand, Indigenous knowledges are powerful for understanding and communicating about the planetary health crisis. Biodiversity loss and climate change can be framed as an outcome of colonisation (rather than simply being caused by 'development' or greenhouse gas emissions) and solutions therefore involve protecting Country and supporting the cultural determinants of health (rather than simply regulating development or decarbonising), with Indigenous land justice and self-determination essential to care for Country (Pascoe & Shukuroglou, 2020; Williams & Sweet, 2021). The mainstream media's inattention to Country and its role as vital life-force in Indigenous peoples' lives makes it complicit in the ongoing colonial process; much research has found the media has perpetuated deficit discourse and fears about Aboriginal and Torres Strait Islander people as violent and destructive (Williams et al., 2017). Protecting planetary health requires strategies for reconnecting and strengthening connections of Aboriginal and Torres Strait Islander peoples to Country and recovering knowledges lying silent – but not lost – in languages, stories and practices (Williams & Sweet, 2021). The Uluru Statement, with its interconnected objectives of Voice, Treaty, Truth, represents a political pathway forward for these cultural determinants of health, and thus also for planetary health and health for all; at the time this chapter was being written, the 2023 referendum for an Aboriginal and Torres Strait Islander Voice to Parliament was being widely discussed in the media and other public spheres, often in ways that reflected racist, colonial ideologies, and circulated misinformation and disinformation. This contributed to the outcome of the failed referendum.

The health impacts of the politics of media and media policy

The media ecosystem

We begin by exploring the media and explaining it as an ecosystem. Ecosystems thinking is dynamic, interconnected and layered. It reflects knowledges and processes of Indigenous people that are holistic, and connect issues and people to each other in systems that produce determinants of health, including cultural, social, commercial and political ones, all of which influence and are influenced by the news and information ecosystem. The concept of the 'news and information ecosystem' encapsulates the complexity and interconnectedness of news and information systems, and the diversity of elements in the ecosystem involved in creating, sharing and using news and information. Within the news and information ecosystem exist a diverse range of media entities, including multinational corporations, such as News Corp and Meta (formerly Facebook), as well as public media organisations, such as NITV, SBS and ABC and not-for-profit media organisations, community-based media, Blak media, and alternative organisations such as the Betoota Advocate and The Juice Media. Media organisations often serve particular sectors and interest groups; for example, *Probono News* was focused on the not-for-profit sector (until its closure, announced in 2023) while the *Australian Financial Review* serves the needs and interests of the business sector, and the *Star Observer* reports for LGBQTIA+SB communities. News and information are produced by a variety of actors, including journalists, writers, photographers, editors, graphic artists, broadcasters, podcasters, digital producers, community members, public health advocates and organisations, film-makers, and satirists, such as those contributing to the Juice Media and its 'Honest Government Ads', and the ABC TV series, *Mad as Hell*. Freelance journalists and independent publishers are also important components of the media sector. Within a single media organisation there may be journalists and other content producers with specific beats or rounds, such as those covering health, politics, business and Indigenous affairs.

In the news and information ecosystem, elements that influence health and wellbeing include community members and organisations, journalists and media organisations, social media participants and companies, and health practitioners, educators and organisations. The ideologies underpinning news and media production are also diverse and influence health and wellbeing, with decolonising and emancipatory processes, on the one hand, and neoliberalism and Whiteness, on the other (Sweet, 2017). Historical forces continue to play out in the ecosystem; *The Guardian*, for example, a progressive global media organisation, has acknowledged its connections to slavery and the social, economic and health disadvantages and violence that perpetrates across generations (Mohdin, 2023).

Spotlight: Power dynamics

Media corporations such as News Corp and Big Tech companies such as Google and Meta are among the most powerful elements of the ecosystem. They also drive and benefit from significant financial profits, visibility, status and political power. They advance the interests of many other commercial determinants of health, including fossil fuels, tobacco, alcohol and gambling industries, all known to be harmful for human and planetary health. The amplification of racism, misinformation and disinformation on platforms, such as Google and Meta, and on media platforms, such as Sky News, often benefits the business model of these companies (Williams & Sweet, 2021). The economic and political power of these companies is enmeshed with the political determinants of the planetary health crisis. That is, Big Tech and dominant media corporations have far more power than not-for-profit and community organisations to influence what information is available to the public, and to shape discourse about certain issues, populations and political processes.

From a public health perspective, the 'commercial determinants of health' are interconnected with political determinants of health, the commercial determinants being for-profit corporations and related entities that seek to make profits (*The Lancet*, 2023) including from their ownership and use of dominant elements of the news and information ecosystem (Williams & Sweet, 2021) as well as of healthcare facilities and prisons (Sweet, 2017; *The Lancet*, 2023). Government policies and processes have enabled inequities in resource allocation and power, favouring corporate interests in ways that undermine the determinants of planetary health (Lacy-Nichols et al., 2022; *The Lancet*, 2023).

Indigenous perspective: Dangerous mining

State and federal governments supported the development of asbestos mining in Western Australia from the 1930s until the 1960s on Banjima Country (Musk et al., 2020). More than 50 years after the closure of the Wittenoom crocidolite (blue asbestos) mine and mill in 1966, it still causes significant illness and premature deaths. Aboriginal people have been disproportionately impacted including by mesothelioma. Traditional Owners are still advocating for their Country to be restored. It is understood as the largest contaminated site in the southern hemisphere (Robinson, 2022).

Public interest journalism

The concept of journalism encompasses a wide range of styles of professional practice, from entertainment news to hyperlocal reporting and public interest journalism, which we define as a type of journalism that gives people the information they need to take part in the democratic process, and that informs and contributes to policy and practice. Further, public interest journalism holds power to account, and amplifies the voices of those who are not well served by the current distribution of power (Croakey Health Media, 2019). Citizen journalism is produced by individuals and organisations who do not identify as traditional journalism practitioners but nonetheless contribute to journalism outcomes and share journalism values. In exploring the news and information ecosystem, it can be helpful to consider public interest journalism as an important determinant of health in and of itself. It seeks to give people the information they need at an individual level to care for their health and at a community level to take part in the democratic process, which seeks and requires informed citizens to make decisions in the interest of planetary health. Public interest journalism is concerned with contributing to engaged and informed communities, and accountable policy making and practice. A collaborative form of public interest journalism is 'social journalism' (Sweet, 2017). This seeks to use the skills of journalism to help meet the needs identified by communities. It can encompass services beyond traditional journalistic content production, including community organising and education. The experience of Croakey Health Media is that public interest journalism can be seen as one of the diverse disciplines of public health.

Public health practitioners and organisations have much to contribute to a sustainable, diverse public interest journalism sector. Many public health practitioners and organisations contribute to the roles of citizen journalism; for example, by live-tweeting conferences or other events. They also write opinion articles for publications, give interviews and tips for stories, as well as directly supporting independent media through subscriptions and funding, or by advocating for media policy to support a more diverse and healthier media sector. Public health practitioners are also involved in the governance and editorial activities of organisations such as Croakey Health Media. Collaborations for media innovation and public interest journalism help meet the needs of under-served communities, and promote planetary health, climate justice and caring for Country.

Let's think

Go to the Croakey Health Media article (2020), 'Save public interest journalism for health', available at: https://www.croakey.org/save-public-interest-journalism-for-health/. Review the three calls for public health action and then:

1   Summarise what doing the three actions means in your own words.
2   Identify a barrier to each of these actions.
3   Who do you think has responsibility, power and position to undertake the actions?
4   What roles might you have in the future where you could contribute to these actions?

Disruption

In 2013, a prominent Australian journalist and academic, Margaret Simons, proclaimed in a book examining the impact of digital disruption upon journalistic practices and the media industry that journalism was living through a 'very exciting but also rather frightening transformation' (Simons, 2013, p. vii). The Internet and the development of digital platforms such as Twitter (now X) meant that the traditional gatekeeper roles of media organisations, as having great power over the selection and presentation of news, had been upended. Some held high hopes that 'democratisation' of the news would flow from citizens being able to take on many of the traditional roles of journalists, undermining the power of media corporations, such as News Corp, and enabling user-driven innovation to better represent diverse communities, as exemplified by the successful @IndigenousX initiative, which has privileged the voices of Aboriginal and Torres Strait Islander peoples and organisations. The development of digital publishing revealed a significant community of interest for the type of coverage that often struggles to capture mainstream news editors' attention, and has enabled the development of greater diversity in media, both in content and structure. But times of disruption bring threats as well as opportunities. In the intervening years, the growing dominance of extractive industries, such as Meta and Google, led to a concentration of power that undermines the economy, innovation, public health and public interest journalism. Outcomes include the contraction and closure of many newsrooms with thousands of journalism job losses, a poorly regulated online environment where anti-health agendas proliferate, and a media ecosystem where corporate agendas continue to dominate, often to the detriment of the public interest and planetary health. A powerful example was when Meta closed community news resource pages during the global COVID-19 pandemic as part of their corporate strategy to resist regulatory pressure (Williams & Sweet, 2021). Likewise, since Elon Musk took over Twitter in 2022, the public interest merits of the platform have been undermined.

In Australia, media policymaking has a long history of supporting dominant corporate media interests. One of the consequences is that corporate media, often representing corporate interests rather than the interests of communities or Country, have undue influence over political processes and outcomes, undermining many of the determinants of planetary health. Longstanding policy recommendations for developing a more diverse and sustainable media ecosystem have not been implemented, although the Albanese Government has committed to changing this dynamic. Much policymaking has been narrowly focused rather than taking whole-of-government approaches to addressing concerns such as the growing problem of 'news deserts', whereby many communities do not have access to reliable, local news sources (see the Public Interest Journalism Initiative, available at: https://piji.com.au/).

Systemic disruption of the news and media ecosystem is needed to transform it into a healthier, more sustainable landscape. As outlined earlier, decolonising methodologies offer a powerful framework for disruption that centres on the health of Country and communities rather than profits of extractive industries. For tens of thousands of years, hundreds of First Nations communities used a knowledge-based economy focused on the production of education, law, entertainment, medicine, spirituality and justice (Sveiby & Skuthorpe, 2006). Knowledges were shared between and across generations; a healthy communications ecosystem was intrinsic to healthy cultures and Country.

Let's do

This activity involves developing a pitch for 'an op-ed article' in a print/online media outlet. Op-ed articles traditionally appeared opposite a newspaper's editorial and are opinion articles. Competition for media space is intense, so prepare your pitch carefully! Consider: (1) WHY you are writing this now; (2) WHAT you hope to achieve; (3) WHO you hope to influence; and (4) HOW to make your argument. Media organisations that publish op-ed articles include ABC, NITV, SBS, Indigenous X, Croakey Health Media, *The Conversation*, and commercial entities such as *The Sydney Morning Herald*. Identify a public health topic to write about, and the media organisation most suited. Develop three bullet points for your pitch, making a strong case for why your article is relevant.

Systems approach

Now we will consider the how colonisation has shaped the media landscape in ways that privilege some interests and undermine others. Colonisation involves patterns of deliberate traumatic assaults, both physical and metaphysical, reaching across generations. These include: the theft and degradation of Country; warfare and violence; legal rights violations; the historical amnesia of the colonisers and settler society versus Aboriginal and Torres Strait Islander peoples' lived experience of colonial history; the dominance of white supremacy and privilege; racism and exclusion; structural violence in policy; and discursive violence, including through the pathologising and deficit-framing of Aboriginal and Torres Strait Islander people (Sweet, 2017). Since colonisation, dominant forms of media have privileged colonial and corporate interests, often undermining rights and humanity of Aboriginal and Torres Strait Islander people, including their rights to care for Country. This was exemplified by *The Bulletin* magazine declaring on its masthead, even into the 1960s, 'Australia for the White Man'. *The Bulletin*, published from 1880 to 2008, was a politically, culturally and socially powerful publication. Concerns about mainstream media's negative coverage of issues affecting Aboriginal and Torres Strait Islander people have been raised over many decades, including by the Royal Commission into Aboriginal Deaths in Custody (Williams et al., 2017). Meanwhile, countless inquiries have drawn attention to the concentrated nature of contemporary media ownership in Australia, and the adverse consequences for policymaking, especially for First Nations peoples and planetary health.

Taking a systems approach helps reveal the web of interconnections between the determinants of health in the news and information ecosystem, threading from the past to the present. It enables us to see threads connecting the commercial, social and cultural determinants of health, and how these create patterns that shape the news and information environment, as well as being shaped by them. For example, industries and interests that undermine health have long used the media as part of strategic efforts to ward off regulation and other public health interventions that threaten their markets and profits. The food industry will promote the importance of individual consumer choice for a healthy diet, which distracts focus from regulatory measures such as clear consumer labelling. They strategically undermine public health evidence and messaging and in turn further their own interests (*The Lancet*, 2023). The political power of such industries undermines social determinants of health. For example, if governments followed the public health evidence and increased taxes on these industries, more public funds could become available for environmental protection, public education, housing and income support – as well as having direct health benefits by reducing fossil fuels, tobacco and alcohol. Likewise, the powerful mining lobby has long undermined cultural determinants of health by opposing and undermining Aboriginal and Torres Strait Islander people's rights to self-determination and protocols and practices for caring for Country. Conversely, collective activism and advocacy by Aboriginal and Torres Strait Islander people and organisations has helped build public and political support for policies that protect Country and cultural sites.

Media organisations themselves can represent the commercial, social and cultural determinants of health in different contexts and situations. For example, public interest journalism can challenge and expose the power of commercial interests, and has over many decades supported public health advocacy and regulation of the tobacco industry. Blak media, community media and public interest journalism organisations that strive to ensure communities are well informed about critical public interest issues and empowered to enact their rights can be seen as positive upstream determinants of health and planetary health by contributing to the accountability of governments and other power-holders. On the other hand, corporate media organisations and Big Tech companies can undermine public health by taking advertising dollars from the purveyors of misinformation and disinformation, undermining planetary health in many ways.

Limelight

From 1952 until 1963, the British Government, supported by the Australian Government, carried out nuclear tests on Aboriginal Country: the Monte Bello Islands off Western Australia, and at Emu Field and Maralinga in South Australia. Aboriginal Country has also been subjected to uranium prospecting, mining and waste dumping. The articles by Urwin (2019) and ICAN Australia (2022) outline the history of uranium mining in Australia and leadership by Aboriginals for a global ban on nuclear weapons. Use these to pitch a related story to a local, national and global media organisation.

Upstream-downstream

Mainstream media health coverage typically privileges the voices of health professionals, especially doctors, and suggests that medical research and healthcare are primarily responsible for the health and wellbeing of populations. In particular, mainstream media tend to focus on hospitals and high-tech interventions rather than prevention and public health. This can distort public and policy debate, so that resources flow fastest to the downstream of healthcare such as hospital beds rather than upstream to where health problems can be prevented, such as health-promoting urban design, housing security and liveable incomes. This focus on healthcare neglects cultural determinants of health, such as self-determination and land rights for First Nations peoples. It also obscures from public and policy debate the importance of the social determinants of health in creating the conditions to enable planetary health. This focus on healthcare also undermines efforts to tackle the commercial determinants of health, by encouraging people to see health as a commodity created by individual behaviour and medical intervention, rather than as a collective good that is created by health-promoting environments and policies that regulate and minimise the impact of harmful corporate interests, such as the fossil fuels, tobacco, gambling, Big Food and alcohol industries.

Public health practitioners are well placed to support and encourage media organisations and journalists to cover the implications of wider policies for planetary health, and to report upon the cultural, social and commercial determinants of health. The Health in All Policies concept provides a framework for interrogating the implications for health and health equity of policies outside the health portfolio; for example, in environmental, industry, social, policing, justice, economic, education, and transport policy. It is especially useful as we face climate disruption and other planetary health crises that demand systemic responses across multiple sectors. Supporting journalists and media organisations to engage with the knowledge of people with lived experience can also help to transform public and policy debates about health. For example, people with lived experience of colonisation, displacement, incarceration, violence, racism, poverty, housing insecurity, food insecurity, exclusion, and climate disruption can help to challenge dominant mainstream narratives about health and wellbeing. It is especially important that the voices and experiences of young people be considered in these contexts.

Spotlight: Advocacy action

Aboriginal and Torres Strait Islander people are on the frontlines of climate action, using collective organising, the law and other public health strategies to protect Country and stop extractive fossil fuels industries. Youth Verdict, a First Nations-led youth organisation in Queensland, took billionaire Clive Palmer to court to challenge his plans for a coal mine in the Galilee basin on human rights grounds. First Nations witnesses gave evidence on Country about how climate change is destroying their cultural rights, through rising sea levels, disrupted seasons and damage to sacred sites. In an historic verdict on 25 November 2022, Queensland Land Court president Fleur Kingham recommended that the Queensland Minister for Environment reject Waratah's application for Environmental Authority and that the Minister for Mining and Resources reject Waratah's Mining Lease application. Check the Youth Verdict website (https://www.youthverdict.org.au/) to find out more about this important case and further developments. Reflect upon why mainstream media has often failed to portray the courage, determination and achievements of First Nations people in working to protect Country, and whose interests have been served in that process?

Global context

In November 2022, Gumbaynggirr nyami Amba-Rose Atkinson joined First Nations Peoples from around the world in Egypt for the 27th United Nations Climate Change Conference (COP27). A researcher at the University of Queensland, Atkinson's PhD study looks at the relationship between Country, climate, and First Nations people's health, and how the knowledge systems of this relationship can and must be embedded in localised and place-based environmental, climate, and health solutions. As well as participating in the conference, Atkinson wrote articles for a #HealthyCOP27 series published by Croakey Health Media in partnership with the Lowitja Institute. Her articles are a powerful example of engaging in public spheres for advocacy, knowledge translation and decolonising. 'To salvage the future of the planet, and humanity, we must challenge existing systems of colonialism, capitalism, and extractivism that fuel climate change,' she wrote. See: https://www.croakey.org/at-cop27-and-beyond-first-nations-voices-and-solutions-must-be-heard-at-all-times-and-at-every-level-of-society/

The health impacts of the politics of misinformation and misinformation policy

Access to information

Access to reliable, relevant and timely information is critical for the health of individuals and communities, as well as for others who also have a role in contributing to planetary health, including policy makers and political decision-makers. As discussed previously, it is useful to see news and information as being in an ecosystem. Ecosystems thinking stimulates critical thinking in layers – for individuals, families and communities, services and systems, the environment and the planet. The news and information ecosystem has the potential to benefit health but is often toxic because of the pervasiveness of misinformation and disinformation.

These closely related concepts are generally distinguished by whether their creation and/or dissemination involved intent. Misinformation refers to false information that is spread, regardless of whether there is intent to mislead, where disinformation is deliberately misleading or biased information, such as propaganda. The news and information ecosystem is especially toxic for individuals and communities who experience misinformation and disinformation expressed through racism, discrimination, hate speech and other forms of violence. It is also important to acknowledge that this toxicity can be intensified for those with intersectional experiences, for example, LGBQTIA+SB communities and First Nations communities. This toxicity reflects regulatory failure and the dominance of corporate interests whose business model makes profits from the dissemination of misinformation and disinformation that not only harms human health and wellbeing but also has wide-ranging adverse consequences for planetary health.

Global context

When a landmark report warned in 2018 that humanity had only 12 years to slash greenhouse gas emissions or face a catastrophic future, only 22 of the 50 biggest newspapers in the United States covered the news. Disasters whose intensity and frequency have been increased by climate change are often reported without climate change even being mentioned. These are just some of many examples of the media's failures in covering the climate crisis. They are some of the reasons that were given to explain the founding of a global media collaboration, Covering Climate Now, which supports media to cover the crisis more systematically and comprehensively. The collaboration supports journalists and media organisations to focus on equity and amplifying the voices of particular communities, including First Nations peoples. It has grown rapidly since its founding in 2019 to become the world's largest media collaborative, with more than 500 news and media partners and 57 countries represented. The collaboration enables content sharing and provides a wealth of tips and resources for covering many related topics, including climate politics, and for addressing climate disinformation and misinformation. According to the founders of Covering Climate Now, 'It is our great misfortune to live at a time when the global peril of climate change coincides with a structural undermining of the media's economic ability to cover a story of this magnitude', as newsroom budgets and staff have been cut. See https://www.cjr.org/special_report/climate-change-media.php

While misinformation and disinformation often are portrayed as 21st Century problems associated with the market dominance of Big Tech, corporate media and other powerful commercial determinants of health, they have long been employed to advance the interests of some groups and undermine the interests of others. For example, the nation state of Australia was built upon the 'white supremacist doctrine' of *terra nullius*, a fiction that was legally maintained until the Mabo decision in 1992 (Watson, 2007, p. 17). This fiction has had a profound impact upon the health and wellbeing of Country, as it was used to justify and enable the dispossession of peoples with the longest history and knowledge of caring for Country. It enabled the degradation of Country through agriculture, mining, urbanisation and other forms of commercial and private development. Decolonising methodologies seek to connect and reconnect humans to Country, through intimate knowledges of Country and of self, with an holistic understanding that healing Country means healing self, and healing self means addressing disconnections colonialism creates from the Country of our ancestors, no matter where we are from.

The separation of people from Country is not only an issue for Indigenous people. This fiction, that people are separate from nature, has underpinned a long legacy of policymaking that has been detrimental for planetary health, whether we consider the decline in biodiversity since colonisation, ongoing damage to cultural sites, or the rising greenhouse gas emissions that are already having significant harmful impacts upon human health and ecosystems at temperature rises that are still far below those already locked in, as a result of historic and ongoing emissions.

Let's do

This activity is to develop your own meaningful Acknowledgement of Country. It brings about critical self-reflection, a health professional capability now in legislation about cultural safety. An Acknowledgement is a cultural protocol for Country and for all on Country. Fill in your details below, informed by some local research and words that flow for you. Say an Acknowledgement each time you undertake actions of significance on the lands of Indigenous peoples.

My name is <add>. I am from people of <add your country/nation> and of <name your> culture. My family came to these lands now known as Australia in the year <add which year> from <add> by <add how and why>. I grew up on the lands of the <name which> people. About my relationship with Aboriginal and Torres Strait Islander Australia – I am <add what it is; for example 'only just learning', or 'on a learning journey and have been for a few years through <add detail>' or 'working in partnerships with <name organisations if appropriate>'.

I acknowledge <local Owners> of the <broader Nation> on whose lands we meet today. I acknowledge ancestors and Elders of the past, and Elders of the present as knowledge holders for these lands.

Let's do

You have been given the opportunity to guest tweet for Croakey Health Media's @WePublicHealth account for a week. Your brief is to investigate how the fossil fuel industry has contributed to misinformation and disinformation about the climate crisis. Identify five articles, from the media or the academic literature, on the topic. Draft a Twitter (now X) thread on each article, with at least five tweets in each thread, summarising each article. After you have drafted these five Twitter threads, draft a sixth thread in which you reflect upon what you have learnt from doing this exercise. Read more about @WePublicHealth at: https://www.croakey.org/wepublichealth/

Marketing and public relations

Changes in the news and information ecosystem in recent years – including the rise of digital platforms and the digital economy – have enabled pervasive marketing of unhealthy products, including alcohol and gambling. The dominant market power of the digital platforms has also been associated with the spread of misinformation and disinformation, as well as harmful systems and ideologies, such as colonialism, neoliberalism and racism. The increasing use of

Artificial Intelligence (AI) across many sectors – including those contributing to the news and information ecosystem – can be expected to exacerbate many of these concerns. These changes are threatening even areas where there have been major advances in health promotion and prevention, such as tobacco control.

Looking back at the history of tobacco control illustrates the importance of proactive public health engagement with news and information ecosystems. Reducing smoking is not only good for the health of people; it is also a planetary health intervention given the wide-ranging environmental harms of tobacco growing, including deforestation and use of fossil fuels. It may seem difficult to believe these days, but, in the past, doctors featured in advertisements promoting cigarettes. Television and radio broadcasts as well as newspapers and magazines once published cigarette advertisements and promotions. Health advocates worked hard over decades to end this pollution of the news and information ecosystem, advocating for regulations to stop such advertising as part of wider tobacco control measures. From the early 1960s onwards, one prominent tobacco control advocate, Dr Nigel Gray, alone wrote to 14 different Ministers for Communication under seven different governments over more than 20 years (Greenhalgh, Scollo, & Winstanley, 2023). In 1971, the Cancer Council produced a groundbreaking series of television commercials featuring high-profile TV actors and comedians parodying popular tobacco advertisements of the time. Tobacco control advocates also worked directly with many journalists, supporting investigations and articles about industry strategies, impacts and political influence, including tits donations to political parties. These activities helped to create political support for tobacco control measures. Between 1973 and 1976, direct cigarette advertising on radio and television was phased out. In 1989, a national ban was introduced on tobacco advertising in print media. The tobacco industry countered by sponsoring sporting and cultural events and organisations – and this was not stopped until 1996. In 2003, Australia signed the World Health Organization Framework Convention on Tobacco Control (WHO FCTC), which defines tobacco advertising and promotion as 'any form of commercial communication, recommendation or action with the aim, effect or likely effect of promoting a tobacco product or tobacco use either directly or indirectly'. It requires that each country shall 'undertake a comprehensive ban on all tobacco advertising, promotion and sponsorship'. More than 90% of the world's population are covered by the treaty, making it one of the most widely embraced treaties in United Nations history.

In pushing for tobacco control measures, health and medical advocates and organisations recognised the importance of engaging with the news and information system in shaping the political determinants of tobacco control, including community attitudes and practices as well as policymaking and laws. They also recognised that tobacco control depended upon reform of that ecosystem itself and the need to for multi-pronged strategies to tackle the commercial determinants of health to address the spread of misinformation and disinformation.

Spotlight: Power dynamics

Interventions promoting digital literacy and health literacy are often suggested as solutions to misinformation and disinformation. The rationale is that equipping people to critically assess the reliability and relevance of news and information will help them to identify and disregard misinformation and disinformation, and make decisions more conducive to health and wellbeing, whether they are voting at elections, doing the grocery shopping or deciding whether to have a particular healthcare intervention. However, this is akin to asking people to put on a Hazmat protective suit when going about their everyday lives, rather than ensuring their environments are safe. The Hazmat approach does not respect the right to a safe, health-promoting news and information environment that is free of misinformation and disinformation; nor does it address inequities whereby some groups, such as young children and older people, are at increased risk. Using an ecosystems model encourages interventions to address the political and commercial determinants of health that result in unsafe news and information environments. This approach recognises that powerful forces – including global corporations, extremist ideologies and malevolent actors – are responsible for the pollution transmitted through digital and physical worlds. Prevention relies upon regulation and systemic, coordinated responses from nation states and global institutions. These can draw upon lessons from 'the public health playbook' that challenge 'the corporate playbook' (Lacy-Nichols et al., 2022).

#RaiseTheAge

The following case study provides an example of how misinformation can drive policymaking that is harmful for Aboriginal and Torres Strait Islander people and communities and undermines the cultural determinants of health. It thus also harms planetary health by undermining the capacity of Aboriginal and Torres Strait Islander people, communities and organisations to care for Country and to share this knowledge between generations and with the general population.

In 2023, the Queensland Labor Government passed laws that are certain to result in more children being incarcerated, with Aboriginal and Torres Strait Islander children most at risk from the new laws. The laws, which were also supported by the Liberal National Party, include overriding the State's Human Rights Act to make breach of bail an offence for children. Children are overwhelmingly not in control of the strategies or resources to achieve bail; with parents, guardians and foster carers, schools and other adults being responsible for children. Research around the world has shown bail conditions are biased to mainstream and not Indigenous community realities. The Queensland laws were passed despite undermining state and national policy agreements aimed at improving the health and wellbeing of Aboriginal and Torres Strait Islander people and stopping such unjust laws. Critics of the laws – who included Aboriginal and Torres Strait Islander health, public health and medical experts, lawyers and human rights advocates – saw them as a political response to alarmist media headlines about youth crime. The passage of these laws is a reminder of the long history of mainstream media in driving punitive 'law and order' responses to crime, rather than encouraging evidence-based investment in communities to prevent crime and provide at-risk young people with care and services rather than carceral responses. Queensland is far from the only jurisdiction to implement such harsh policies that disproportionately affect Aboriginal and Torres Strait Islander children and young people.

For decades, Aboriginal and Torres Strait Islander communities and organisations, working together with public health, medical, legal and human rights organisations, have been advocating for law reform to raise the age of criminal responsibility from 10 to 14 and to promote investment in cultural programs and initiatives for children and their families and communities. #RaiseThe-Age is a hashtag that has been used in effective advocacy campaigns in the mainstream, community and social media. In 2022, the nation's Attorney-General released a draft report that had recommended Commonwealth, State and Territory governments should in 2020 raise the minimum age of criminal responsibility to 14 years of age. The ongoing incarceration of young children when evidence-based alternatives are available (Trevitt, 2022) is a reminder of how power dynamics and misinformation in the news and information ecosystem play out, disadvantaging those with the least power and political capital, and perpetuating the legacy of colonisation. The criminalisation of children and young people – who often are experiencing the effects of systemic bias, trauma and poverty – is a reminder of the importance of decolonising frameworks in working to transform these power dynamics. The #JustJustice project supported by Croakey Health Media is an example of a collaborative journalism project that was informed by decolonising methodology. It provided a powerful counter narrative to mainstream media headlines, and drew upon the expertise of Aboriginal and Torres Strait Islander communities and public health experts (Williams et al., 2017).

The activity below explores how misinformation and disinformation contribute to harmful policy outcomes for asylum seekers and refugees, at a time when the planetary health crisis is increasing their number and vulnerability.

Let's think

Misinformation and disinformation have a profound impact upon the wellbeing of asylum seekers and refugees, to the extent that the United Nations High Commissioner for Refugees (UNHCR) has developed resources for addressing these concerns: https://www.unhcr.org/innovation/wp-content/uploads/2022/02/Factsheet-4.pdf

Using this fact sheet and the prompts below, identify an example of misinformation or disinformation undermining health and wellbeing of asylum seekers and refugees.

	Example and type of misinformation	*Source/s of misinformation*	*Motivation for misinformation*	*Potential impacts*	*Public health responses*
Source X					

Spotlight: Advocacy action

It is unfortunate that the two separate initiatives Close the Gap and Closing the Gap are often confused, including in media reporting and by health professionals and the wider community. Close the Gap is a campaign by Aboriginal and Torres Strait Islander community-controlled peak bodies, human rights organisations and other non-Indigenous non-government organisations for health equity through a strengths-based approach, highlighting the importance of the cultural determinants of health. On the other hand, Closing the Gap is the governments' framework, which, since 2008, has reported annually on targets but has never yet fully achieved these. Only since 2019 have governments worked in partnership with Aboriginal and Torres Strait Islander organisations through the Coalition of Peaks, which represents more than 80 Aboriginal and Torres Strait Islander community-controlled peak organisations and members. Advocates have raised concerns about the dominance and impacts of governments' use of deficits-based language and framing in Closing the Gap. This deficit framing, amplified throughout the news and information ecosystem, has been a key strategy of colonisation and has been powerful in undermining political and public support for Aboriginal and Torres Strait Islander people's leadership. The ramifications of this framing – a form of misinformation – have been far-reaching and detrimental to planetary health. It has taken western knowledge systems and politics hundreds of years to begin to understand the importance of using Indigenous knowledge systems for planetary health.

Decolonising

Indigenous organisations and peoples globally have urged researchers, policymakers and communities to engage with decolonising methodologies across diverse fields, including planetary health, public health and the media. Decolonising methodologies enable and drive changes to systems, structures and norms in support of planetary health. Decolonising is a dynamic process that cannot be taken alone or in isolation; it requires a community-wide effort that understands people as part of wider systems and ecosystems. It requires that systems, structures, practices and norms privilege the voices and knowledges of First Nations peoples, and support self-determination and the cultural determinants of health. Decolonising also requires non-Indigenous people to develop their capacity to work in ways that support, rather than undermine, self-determination of First Nations peoples and the cultural determinants of health. This requires changes in systems and structures across all settings, from education and training to workplaces and communities. It requires us all to engage in systems thinking that recognises everyone has a role in contributing to healthier, and more diverse, news and information ecosystems where misinformation and disinformation are the exception rather than the norm. This cannot happen without a rebalancing of power and political dynamics so that ownership and control no longer reside in the hands of powerful corporations, but in the hands of communities, and most especially First Nations communities. Efforts to decolonise news and information ecosystems therefore require systemic efforts involving multiple actors and systems.

Indigenous perspective

Indigenous peoples worldwide have clear protocols for sharing news and information – knowledge transfer. Wiradjuri people, for example, consider the impacts of knowledges, including news and information, in the context of seven generations. The aim is to understand where knowledges emanate from and are transferred to, ensuring they cause no harm, contribute to unity, and protect Country. These principles are reflected in international Indigenous Data Sovereignty and Governance statements; they are also identifiable in Australian health and medical ethics guidelines for research, and they align with media codes of ethics. These protocols are critical for tackling misinformation and disinformation, as has been evident during the COVID-19 pandemic. To role-model excellence, the Lowitja Institute and Croakey Health Media produced *Profiling Excellence: Indigenous Knowledge Translation* (Williams, 2021).

Let's finish

In 2019, Professor Bronwyn Carlson, from the Department of Indigenous Studies at Macquarie University on the lands of the Wattamattagal clan of the Darug nation in Sydney, was the keynote speaker for the Association of Internet Researchers (AoIR) conference in Meaanjin/Brisbane. Her research investigates how the lives of Indigenous peoples are increasingly impacted by digital technologies and especially social media. After her presentation highlighting some of the harms and benefits of social media, an audience member asked Professor Carlson whether she would pull the plug on social media, if she could.

Professor Carlson answered in the affirmative, writing in a later reflection:

> It is not that I do not recognise the benefits of social media; clearly, there are many. I just think we can do better. We need to unhinge ourselves from the idea that social media in its current form is here to stay and must remain just the way it is now.
>
> I wonder what a global communication tool might look like if it was based on Indigenous ways of knowing, doing and being in the world. Imagine a global communication network that was monitored with care and empathy as opposed to hate, violence and controversy. Imagine if such a platform was regulated by real people and there was accountability to those who were impacted by anything untoward.
>
> Imagine a network based on social justice, equity and all those aspirations that are so often attacked on social media in its current form. Imagine a social media whose interests lie in educating, imparting knowledge equitably, as well as incorporating the humour of life. Imagine a universal network of communication whose underlying principles reflect Indigenous philosophies rather than rampant and unrestrained capitalism.
>
> (Carlson, 2022)

Let's take up Professor Carlson's challenge and imagine a news and information ecosystem that reflects Indigenous philosophies, supports caring for Country and communities, and that provides a safe, respectful space for sharing news and knowledge, and for holding power-holders to account. And imagine that it does this in a purposeful way to support communities, governments and others through escalating climate disruption, with a focus on planetary health for all.

Summary

In this chapter we used decolonising methodologies to outline distinctive features of the Australian news and information ecosystem, political determinants of health, and the relationship between misinformation and disinformation and planetary health.

After studying this chapter, you should be able to apply a decolonising methodologies to:

- *Understand the distinctive features of the Australian media ecosystem and the global context.* This chapter outlined elements of decolonising methodologies such as identifying strategies of colonisation, critical self-reflection, respect for self-determination of Indigenous peoples, and the importance of the cultural determinants of health, including caring for Country, for planetary health.
- *Critique the media landscape, including historical, corporate, cultural and systemic ideologies.* This chapter illustrated how decolonising methodologies could be applied to analysis of the Australian media ecosystem, to illuminate how it is dominated by ideologies such as White supremacy, embedded racism and destruction of Country's health. On the other hand, independent and Blak media enact emancipatory ideologies, such as decolonising.
- *Analyse the impacts of misinformation and disinformation on planetary health.* This chapter discussed the pervasiveness of misinformation and disinformation, giving examples of how this harms planetary health. We identified the dominant market power of Big Tech as a critical concern for planetary health, while also highlighting misinformation and disinformation as integral to the colonial project.
- *Critically synthesise how public health can contribute to a healthier media landscape.* This chapter identified public interest journalism as an important determinant of health in and of itself. It seeks to give people the information they need at an individual level to care for

their health and at a community level to take part in the democratic process, which seeks and requires informed citizens to make decisions in the interest of planetary health. We discussed how the public health community can contribute to public interest journalism and a healthier media landscape in many ways.

Tutorial exercises

1   Review the Seed Mob website: https://www.seedmob.org.au/ and identify three ways that you can support this organisation.
2   Read this article at Croakey Health Media (2021): 'New report targets 12 "super spreaders" of COVID-19 misinformation', available at: https://www.croakey.org/new-report-targets-12-super-spreaders-of-covid-19-misinformation/ What are three suggestions for addressing political determinants of planetary health?
3   Examine the latest Reuters Institute Digital News Report https://www.digitalnewsreport.org/. This investigates global trends in digital news production and consumption; the political determinants of planetary health are not named as such in the report but use it to identify three political and commercial determinants of health and three ways public health practitioners can address these, presented as a briefing to the Public Health Association of Australia.

Further reading

Close the Gap. Available at: https://humanrights.gov.au/our-work/aboriginal-and-torres-strait-islander-social-justice/projects/close-gap-indigenous-health

Coalition of Peaks. Available at: https://coalitionofpeaks.org.au/

Croakey Health Media. Archive of articles on public interest journalism. Available at: https://www.croakey.org/category/media-and-health/public-interest-journalism/

Croakey Health Media. (2017–2023). Submissions. Available at: https://www.croakey.org/about-croakey-health-media/croakey-submissions/

Indigenous Data Sovereignty and Governance. Available at: https://www.lowitja.org.au/icms_docs/328550_data-governance-and-sovereignty.pdf

Sweet, M. (2019). Health sector joins the push for regulatory crackdown on Facebook et al. Croakey Health Media, 27 February. Available at: https://www.croakey.org/health-sector-joins-the-push-for-regulatory-crackdown-on-facebook-et-al/

Sweet, M., Williams, M., Armstrong, R., & McInerney, M. (2021). The pandemic and public interest journalism: Crisis, survival – and rebirth? In M. Lewis, E. Govender, & K. Holland (eds), *Communicating COVID-19: Interdisciplinary perspectives*. London: Palgrave Macmillan, pp. 21–40.

Sweet, M. A., Williams, M., Armstrong, R., Mohamed, J., Finlay, S. M., & Coopes, A. (2020). Converging crises: Public interest journalism, the pandemic and public health. *Public Health Research and Practice*, 30(4), e3042029.

Zuboff, S. (2019). *The age of surveillance capitalism: The fight for a human future at the new frontier of power*. London: Profile Books.

References

Ahpra & National Boards. (2020). A strategy for embedding cultural safety into the health system launching tomorrow. Press release. Available at: https://www.ahpra.gov.au/News/2020-02-26-strategy-for-embedding-cultural-safety.aspx

Bailey, J., Blignault, I., Carriage, C., Demassi, K., Joseph, T. ...& Williams, M. (2020). We are working for our people: Growing and strengthening the Aboriginal and Torres Strait Islander health workforce.

Lowitja Institute. Available at: https://www.lowitja.org.au/content/Image/Career_Pathways_Report_ Working_for_Our_People_2020.pdf

Carlson, B. (2022). Online lessons from Indigenous knowledges. Croakey Health Media. 19 January. Available at: https://www.croakey.org/online-lessons-from-indigenous-knowledges/

Croakey Health Media. (2019). Croakey Health Media Strategic Plan, 2019–2022. Available at: https:// www.croakey.org/wp-content/uploads/2020/05/StrategicPlan_22May2020-1-1.pdf

Croakey Health Media. (2020). Save public interest journalism for health. 1 December. Available at: http s://www.croakey.org/save-public-interest-journalism-for-health/

Croakey Health Media. (2021). New report targets 12 'super spreaders' of COVID-19 misinformation. Available at: https://www.croakey.org/new-report-targets-12-super-spreaders-of-covid-19-misinformation/

Fredericks, B., & Adams, K. (2011). Decolonising action research. *ALAR: Action Learning and Action Research Journal*, 17(2), 2–11. http://search.informit.com.au.ezproxy2.library.usyd.edu.au/docum entSummary;dn=463074843913796;res=IELHSS

Fredericks, B., & Legge, D. (2011). Revitalizing Health for All: International Indigenous Representative Group. Learning from the experience of comprehensive primary health care in Aboriginal Australia: A commentary on three projects. Lowitja Institute. Available at: https://www.lowitja.org.au/page/services/ resources/health-services-and-workforce/service-solutions/Revitalizing-Health-for-All

Greenhalgh, E. M., Scollo, M. M., & Winstanley, M. H. (2023). Tobacco in Australia: Facts and issues. Cancer Council Victoria. Available at: https://www.tobaccoinaustralia.org.au/home.aspx.

ICAN Australia. (2022). Statement from people impacted by nuclear testing. ICAN Australia. 23 June. Available at: https://icanw.org.au/statement-nuclear-testing/

Lacy-Nichols, J., Marten, R., Crosbie, E., & Moodie, R. (2022). The public health playbook: ideas for challenging the corporate playbook. *The Lancet*, 10(7), e1067–e1072. https://doi.org/10.1016/ S2214-109X(22)00185-1

Mohdin, A. (2023). Guardian owner apologises for founders' links to transatlantic slavery. *The Guardian*, 29 March. Available at: https://www.theguardian.com/news/2023/mar/28/guardian-owner-apologi ses-founders-transatlantic-slavery-scott-trust

Musk, A. W., Reid, A., Olsen, N., Hobbs, M., Armstrong, B., Franklin, P., Hui, J., Layman, L., Merler, E., & Brims, F. (2020). The Wittenoom legacy. *International Journal of Epidemiology*, 49(2), 467–476. https://doi.org/10.1093/ije/dyz204

Pascoe, B., & Shukuroglou, V. (2020). *Loving Country: A guide to sacred Australia*. Hardie Grant Travel.

Robinson, T. (2022). Traditional Owners reignite debate on stalled plans to clean up asbestos waste at Wittenoom. *ABC News*, 11 October. Available at: https://www.abc.net.au/news/2022-10-11/wittenoom -asbestos-ghost-town-calls-to-restore-area/101504342

Simons, M. (2013). Introduction. In M. Simons (ed.), *What's next in journalism? New media entrepreneurs tell their stories*. Scribe, pp. vii–xvii.

Sveiby, K., & Skuthorpe, T. (2006). *Treading lightly: The hidden wisdom of the world's oldest people*. Crows Nest, NSW: Allen & Unwin. Sweet, M. (2017). Acknowledgement: A social journalism research project relating to the history of lock hospitals, lazarets and other forms of medical incarceration of Aboriginal and Torres Strait Islander people. Thesis, University of Canberra.

Sweet, M. (2022). The crisis in regional journalism: Why it's a big health concern, and some suggested solutions. Croakey Health Media, 2 February. Available at: https://www.croakey.org/the-crisis-in-re gional-journalism-why-its-a-big-health-concern-and-some-suggested-solutions/

The Lancet. (2023). Commercial determinants of health. *The Lancet*. Available at: https://www.thelancet. com/series/commercial-determinants-health

Trevitt, S. (2022,). New report shows the way for governments wanting to stop crime and improve children's lives. Croakey Health Media, 13 October. Available at: https://www.croakey.org/new-report-shows-the-way-for-governments-wanting-to-stop-crime-and-improve-childrens-lives/

Urwin, J. (2019). Uranium mines harm Indigenous people – so why have we approved a new one? *The Conversation*, 6 May. Available at: https://theconversation.com/uranium-mines-harm-indigenous-peop le-so-why-have-we-approved-a-new-one-116262

Walker, R. (2004). Transformative strategies in Indigenous education: A study of decolonisation and positive social change: The Indigenous Community Management Program. Thesis, Curtin University, WA. http://handle.uws.edu.au:8081/1959.7/678

Watson, I. (2007). Settled and unsettled spaces: Are we free to roam? In A. Moreton-Robinson (ed.), *Sovereign subjects: Indigenous sovereignty matters*. New York: Routledge, pp. 1–18.

Williams, M. (ed.). (2021). Profiling excellence: Indigenous knowledge translation. Lowitja Institute. Available at: https://www.lowitja.org.au/page/services/resources/health-policy-and-systems/knowledge-translation/profiling-excellence—indigenous-knowledge-translation

Williams, M., Finlay, S. M., Sweet, M., & McInerney, M. (2017). #JustJustice: Rewriting the roles of journalism in Indigenous health. *Australian Journalism Review*, 39(2), 107–118. https://search.informit.org/doi/10.3316/informit.360484852967858

Williams, M., & Sweet, M. (2021). Healing: Big Tech as a public health crisis. In P. Lewis & J. Guiao (eds), *The Public Square Project: Reimagining our digital future*. Melbourne: Melbourne University Press, pp. 156–168.

Part III

Political Determinants of Our Environment

6 Food and Farming

Kerri-Anne Gill and Katherine Cullerton

World hunger and starvation have everything to do with politics. Political conflicts, insufficient responses to natural disasters, corrupt political institutions, and inequalities in income and education constitute what public health practitioners call the 'root' causes of hunger and malnutrition

(Marion Nestle, *Eat Drink Vote*, 2013)

Learning objectives

After studying this chapter, you should be able to:

1   Understand how governments influence food systems and planetary health.
2   Identify key actors in Australian food policy, their interests, and the ways they influence policy agendas and outcomes.
3   Assess the health impacts of different policy priorities for food and nutrition.
4   Understand the major challenges and opportunities for farmers.
5   Compare the breadth of policy domains that impact farming communities.
6   Identify the interaction between food production and planetary health, and the political influences on this relationship.

Snapshot

After the Second World War, the world's population began to rise at an unprecedented rate. By the 1960s, there was a concerted global effort to meet growing demand for food by increasing production through what became known as the Green Revolution. This encompassed a combination of higher-yielding crop varieties, increased inputs of fertilisers and pesticides, farm specialisation in single commodities, and the use of increasingly complex machinery run on fossil fuels. The spread of Green Revolution technologies was supported by an economic regime that prioritised the interests of funders and removed barriers to free trade (McMichael, 2004). Free markets advocates argued that consumers could enjoy a plentiful supply of goods produced at the lowest cost anywhere in the world if trade barriers were removed and global trade and competition were encouraged (Friedman, 1962).

Today's reality is quite different. More people than ever are going hungry with over three billion people unable to afford a healthy diet in 2022 (FAO et al., 2022). Agricultural policies incentivise the overproduction of cereals at the expense of other nutritionally-important foods, such as vegetables, legumes, nuts and seeds (FAO et al., 2022) while around 30% of all food produced is wasted (UNEP, 2021). Non-communicable diseases now account for around three-quarters of deaths globally, with poor diets being a major cause, along with tobacco use and

DOI: 10.4324/9781003315490-11

alcohol consumption (WHO, 2022). Meanwhile global food systems cause a third of the greenhouse gas emissions driving catastrophic climate change (Crippa et al., 2021). There have been many calls for food system transformation (see, e.g., FAO et al., 2021; IFPRI, 2021; IPES-Food, 2016) but, unfortunately the political will for change around the world is limited.

Let's begin

Good nutrition is essential for health. Conversely, poor nutritional status is linked to the ever-growing rates of non-communicable diseases and obesity that we see in Australia and other countries around the world. Ample evidence exists describing this growing problem but also the solutions that will help mitigate nutrition-related diseases. Despite this, we see limited interest from the Australian government in adopting recommended policies. While there are many reasons policy change does not occur in this area, one key contributor to the limited action is the political practices undertaken by the food industry to maintain the status quo. In the first section of this chapter, we will explore these political practices and the impact they have on the food system in Australia. We begin by addressing the role of food systems in the rise of non-communicable diseases and the politics surrounding government action, or inaction, to address the root causes. We then explore the topic of food insecurity and some of the issues and options for addressing it. In the second section of this chapter, we turn our attention to the people who grow our food and the communities in which they live and work. Australian farmers are among the least subsidised in the Organisation for Economic Co-operation and Development (OECD) and have operated for decades in a policy environment that promotes high yields, production efficiency, and the supply of agricultural commodities to export markets. We will question the extent to which this supports public health goals of aligning production with dietary guidelines and ensuring a sustainable supply of affordable, healthy food. We will consider the policies and politics of farming from a local through to a global level. In doing so, we will first explore the needs and challenges of farming communities and how government policy choices affect the health of those communities. We will then explore the relationships between agriculture, environmental health and climate. We will consider what the Australian Government is doing to both limit and respond to climate impacts in the agriculture sector, and how farmers are working to influence climate policy.

The health impacts of the politics of food and food policy

The food environment

Non-communicable diseases (NCDs), such as cancer and heart disease, are the leading cause of illness and death in Australia. The food and drinks we consume have become the leading behavioural risk factor for developing NCDs worldwide. In particular, high consumption of ultra-processed food containing high amounts of sugar, salt and trans fats, as well as low consumption of healthy foods, for example, fruits and vegetables, nuts and pulses have led to this health crisis. This situation is so dire that we have fewer than 1% of Australians consuming a diet consistent with recommendations for healthy eating in national guidelines (NHMRC, 2013). Importantly, the ever-increasing rise of NCDs is not inevitable. Improving the diets of populations could prevent 20% of deaths globally (Branca et al., 2019). It's tempting to blame individuals for poor eating habits or assume that health education is the key to improving diets. However, we need to remember that the majority of the population is surrounded by an environment that supports the consumption of unhealthy food products. This makes choosing unhealthier options the easy choice much of the time.

> **Let's think**
>
> Food environments impact on food choices in a number of ways, including: which food is available to purchase, how much it costs, how easily you can access retailers to purchase food, whether you have facilities for preparing food, and how often you are exposed to marketing that reminds you to purchase and consume certain foods. *How does your food environment influence your food choices?*

Food environments, particularly unhealthy food environments, are influenced by external factors including government policies that support the production, retailing and marketing of ultra-processed foods. Some of these policies are very clear, such as agricultural policies that support the agricultural sector to grow high yield 'cash crops'. However, other polices are less obvious. These include government decisions not to adopt policies that might protect the public but harm businesses, for example, not implementing a tax on sugary drinks. Research has demonstrated that addressing external factors that affect the food environment is the most effective strategy for improving the health of a population.[1] However, adopting and implementing these measures require governments to intervene via laws and regulations that directly target the drivers of unhealthy food environments. This can be challenging for many governments, including the Australian Government, as it means taking on corporate power and sometimes this position will clash with the governing party's own ideology. This ongoing tension between the health of the population and corporate power has meant many of the strategies recommended to address the drivers of poor food environments have not been adopted in Australia. One of these drivers is the wide availability of unhealthy food options (usually at the expense of healthy options) often at very cheap prices. Another is the industry's use of marketing tactics via the media, social media and billboards that constantly remind people to consume unhealthy products. It is hard to make a healthy choice in this environment.

The food industry

Significant benefits can accrue from improving our food environments. This includes not only health benefits but also financial benefits. Increasing rates of NCDs impose a significant economic burden on taxpayers through costs to the healthcare system as well as reduced taxation receipts to governments due to reduced employee productivity because of ill-health (Crosland et al., 2019). However, there is a group who stands to lose if governments were to tackle the drivers of unhealthy food environments, namely, the food industry. In particular, companies producing ultra-processed foods. For this group, maintaining the status quo to ensure their products continue to sell at the same level (or creating conditions to further increase sales) is their priority. To make sure this occurs, they engage in sophisticated political practices ranging from direct lobbying, which includes meeting politicians and providing donations to parties, to more indirect activities, such as creating a sense of broad support for the industry position through seemingly independent front groups (fake grassroots organisations). By using these strategies, they are able to disseminate narratives that position the regulation of unhealthy foods as an unnecessary solution to nutrition issues like obesity. And, therefore, nothing changes.

Spotlight: Power dynamics

The National Food Plan that never eventuated...

Ideally when thinking about food systems policy, we should consider:

- the supply and demand for food
- the supply chain from producers to consumers
- the food environment that drives consumer choice, and knowledge, attitudes and behaviours.

However, this sort of multi-sector approach is very challenging as there are many vested interests wanting to shape food and nutrition policy.

Illustrating this challenge is the 2013 Australian National Food Plan which never came to fruition. It is helpful to consider how the Plan came to be and what led to its demise. Back in 1992, the declaration of the International Conference on Nutrition required national governments to develop National Plans of Action for Nutrition. They specified that the plans should be inter-sectoral, placing nutrition in the context of broader food system influences on consumption, and involving all relevant government departments, including trade, agriculture and health. This declaration coincided with the release of Australia's first and only nutrition policy. While this policy was lauded for its comprehensiveness, it received limited financial support from the government for implementation.

Since that time, advocates had been calling for a new food and nutrition policy. The chance came when the Labor Government was re-elected in 2010 and announced that it was developing a National Food Plan that would 'integrate all aspects of food policy by looking at the whole food chain, from the paddock to the plate'. However, the process for developing the policy was marred from the start. The Working Group established was heavily 'stacked' by the agriculture and food industry sector. Of the 13 members of the Working Group, 10 were powerful stakeholders from the commercial food and agricultural sector; there was one consumer representative and one health representative. Simultaneously, outside of the Working Group, food industry stakeholders were collaborating with each other, and with government, in developing their vision for the plan. Unfortunately, no such coordinated strategy was occurring from public health stakeholders. Consequently, the National Food Plan started with the intention of being an integrated national food policy, but quickly changed into an industry-focused policy in which both health and environmental sustainability were side-lined. However, in the end, politics trumped all. After the National Food Plan was released, a federal election was held which the Labor Government lost and the new Liberal–National Coalition came to power. The new government supported a neoliberal approach they believed would deliver benefits without government interference. As a result, the National Food Plan was quickly shelved.

For more on this case study, see Carey et al. (2016).

As demonstrated in our Spotlight box, another challenge to the adoption of evidence-based policy to improve food environments is the role of ideology within ruling political parties. Political ideology includes beliefs about whether the responsibility for health lies with the individual or with society, and whether the government has a right, or even a responsibility, to intervene in individual behaviour and commercial activity to protect and promote the public good (Cohen et al., 2000). Ideological arguments that often factor during discussions of public health policies often pit the role of government to intervene to protect the health of its citizens against the right of individuals to make their own choices. In Australia, our conservative parties tend to prefer not to intervene and to allow personal responsibility when it comes to public health policy, whereas progressive parties are more likely to intervene (Cicchini et al., 2021). This can result in long periods of limited policy change when a particular party is in power such as when the conservative coalition parties were in power in Australia for a decade from 2013 to 2022.

Global context: The tactics of transnational food companies globally

The rising rates of NCDs seen in Australia are mirrored all around the world. Rising rates of NCDs driven by increasing consumption of ultra-processed foods is occurring not only in high-income countries but also in low- and middle-income countries. And the drivers are the same: food environments that do not support healthy choices. These are promoted by transnational companies that use every means possible, including legal, regulatory, and societal, to create and protect an environment that is favourable to selling their products in a competitive marketplace.

Around the world, these political practices have been documented: lobbying government officials, providing political donations, media campaigns to influence the public, co-opting nutrition experts in order to influence dietary advice given to the public and to promote an image of their products as nutritious, attacking critics which can include lawsuits, developing front groups to advocate for their products and to lobby against any suggested policy changes which harm sales. This concerted effort has resulted in the continued growth of transnational food and beverage companies and the increased global consumption of their products particularly in low- and middle-income countries. Unfortunately, this has also resulted in rapid increases in overweight and obesity as well as NCDs which have disproportionately affected low- and middle-income countries.

For more on this topic, see Nestle (2002).

Food systems

We have been exploring the role of unhealthy food environments and the drivers of these environments that lead to poor health. We now turn to another source of poor health in Australia – unhealthy food security systems and the political determinants underpinning them. Australia is one of the richest countries in the world, yet we have a growing problem of food insecurity. Food insecurity is when people lack regular access to enough safe and nutritious food for normal growth and development and an active and healthy life (FAO et al., 2022). The causes of food insecurity lie largely outside the influence of the health sector and relate to poverty and financial hardship. However, the health consequences are serious and substantial. When food security systems don't work, it often impacts on the most vulnerable.

Let's do

What policies could governments adopt to tackle the issue of food insecurity? Is it better to focus on the causes of food insecurity, or try to address the effects? One example of how food insecurity is being addressed in Australia is through the rise of food relief, often provided in the form of 'food banks'. *Find information about food banks to understand how they are financed and operate.*

Food banks are charities that rely mostly on donated food waste/surplus from food retailers or hospitality venues that they then give to people in need. While it is admirable that charities exist to help those in need, it is important to consider that the existence of these organisations can reinforce the withdrawal of the government from welfare provision. Also, there can be a sense of shame and stigma attached to food banks for those who use them (Booth & Pollard, 2020). Finally, questions are raised as to whether food banks prevent food insecurity occurring in the future. It is important to remember in this debate that we do have enough food in Australia to feed our entire population, but access and the right to that food are the issues (Caraher & Furey, 2018).

Let's think

As government pulls back from intervening in food security policies, there will be more families going without food and using food banks. This raises questions about the appropriateness of these charity organisations as a solution to food security in the long term. Do you think food banks should be used as a solution to food insecurity? Why, or why not?

While for many Australians food insecurity is caused by a lack of financial access, in some remote areas the biggest challenge is physical access to food. An example is what occurs in the north of Australia when 'the Wet' comes, that is, when summer rains fall, particularly in the Northern Territory and northern Queensland. These rains come every year between December and March, and every year roads going into remote Aboriginal communities are cut off. This means that food needs to be air-lifted or transported by barge to reach these communities at considerable cost, which the community pays for with more expensive food prices in the store. For years, communities in these regions have been calling on governments to fix the roads to ensure a more stable supply of food. However, as these communities are so small, they have very little power to influence policy change and therefore limited action has occurred to improve the roads.

Indigenous perspective: Leadership in food retailing from remote Aboriginal communities

Sometimes when the political will to support healthy food environments is not there, communities can choose to take action themselves. This is what occurred in some remote Aboriginal communities in the Northern Territory. Led by the Arnhem Land Progress Association (ALPA), an Aboriginal-run retail and economic development organisation, a decision was made to change the stores to improve the health of the community. This aligned with ALPA's vision to be concerned not only with the economic growth of the organisation and the social development of communities, but also with the health of their communities. With this in mind, the ALPA Board worked in collaboration with researchers to implement strategies to improve healthy options in their stores and to dissuade customers from purchasing unhealthy options. This initiative resulted in dramatic improvements. In 12 weeks across 10 stores, they sold 1.8 tonnes less sugar, sales of unhealthy drinks fell by 8.4%, money spent on health drinks increased, and the business performance of the stores was not affected. This initiative provides important lessons for all retail stores, and for policymakers, across Australia.

For more on this case study, see Brimblecombe, et al. (2020).

The health impacts of the politics of farming and farming policy

As the major source of food and therefore nutrition for global populations, the agriculture sector plays a key role in human health. It also has significant impacts on planetary health, and is in turn critically dependent on the Earth's natural systems. In the remainder of this chapter, we will consider policies and politics related to farming and their impacts on health – the health of individuals, communities, and the planet. We will encounter a range of different interest groups and their policy priorities. These span individuals and families seeking a stable supply of affordable, healthy food, public health advocates concerned with the nutritional qualities of the food supply and the environmental impacts of farming, commercial agribusinesses and agricultural investors seeking economic returns, and governments tasked with collecting tax revenue, tempering demands on taxpayer funds, and promoting exports to offset the nation's imports. Of course, there are also the interests of the farmers themselves. Farmers' interests are as diverse as their farming enterprises, varying by the farm sector, location, size, history, farming methods, financial and other resources, and the personal vision of the farmer. Farmers ultimately decide what they produce on their land, which methods they use, and to whom they sell what they produce. We will begin by looking locally at issues that affect farmers and their communities. Then we will step back and explore the bigger issues related to climate and how this impacts farming.

Community

The food we eat is produced across a variety of landscapes. Unless you grow your own food in your backyard or a community garden, the majority of your fresh food and the ingredients for processed food will come from distant, rural areas. This is because farmers generally depend on large expanses of fertile land to produce food and other commodities like animal feed. Generally, these large expanses of land are not seen in urban areas as zoning policies prioritise other land uses such as housing, retail, roads, schools, and so on. This leads to higher land values and causes land to be divided into smaller parcels less suited to large-scale farming.

Let's think

In Australia, the decision to zone land for different uses is made by local governments in line with state government land use planning laws and the perceived needs of the community. Population growth can put pressure on councils to rezone rural land for urban development. Property developers profit from developing and selling this land, so it is in their interest to encourage councils to release more land for development. Farmers also have an incentive to sell their land on the urban periphery to developers, since farming often provides limited income for physically demanding work, whereas selling their land for development can attract a substantial pay-out. Do you think peri-urban land should be protected from urban expansion so it can be used for food production? Why, or why not?

For a case study, see James (2014).

The distance between where food is produced and where it is consumed has implications for the nutritional qualities of the food, the environmental impacts of long supply chains, and the accessibility of infrastructure, goods and services to farming communities. We considered nutrition earlier in this chapter and will explore environmental impacts of food and farming systems a little later. For now, let's focus on the health impacts of remoteness on farmers and farming communities.[2] Imagine having to drive hours or even days to get to shops, a doctor or dentist, a hospital or a government service. This is the reality for many farmers who live and work on large, remote farms and livestock stations. For nearly a century, people in remote locations have relied on services like the Royal Flying Doctor Service for medical care and School of the Air for education. More recently, improvements in telecommunication technologies have provided new possibilities in areas, such as telehealth, online learning, and social and business communications. This has enormous potential to improve physical and mental health, reduce social isolation, and influence other determinants of health, such as education and income generation. For farmers to benefit from these technologies, the supporting infrastructure must be in place. Who should provide it? Should governments invest taxpayer funds to build and maintain infrastructure that benefits people in sparsely populated areas? Should businesses be required to provide services to farmers, regardless of where they live? Should farmers living in more remote locations have to pay extra for the same services available at lower cost to people living in urban areas? The answers to these questions depend on the values policymakers assign to different policy outcomes.

Let's do

The way policy actors evaluate needs and policy options depends very much on their values and goals. Consider the following list of goals for providing infrastructure to farming communities and rank them from most to least important. Compare your ranking to those of your classmates and discuss any differences.

- Ensuring everyone has access to the basic essential services.
- Giving everyone the same standard of service regardless of where they live.
- Minimising infrastructure spending so taxes can be lowered.
- Investing in infrastructure that will endure well into the future.
- Making users pay to procure services that meet their own needs, preferences, and budget.
- Providing businesses with opportunities to supply services for profit.
- Ensuring any taxpayer-funded investments are fully costed and provide an adequate return.
- Or something else?

For more on the values and belief systems of policy advocates, see *The Common Cause Handbook* (Holmes et al., 2012).

As highlighted earlier, the ideological positions of different political parties affect their policy preferences. This includes the positions they adopt on how essential services and infrastructure should be provided. In the early 1990s, Australian governments chose to privatise several major public entities encompassing services such as telecommunications, banking and aviation. This yielded short-term financial gains for the government but led to complaints of reduced service and increased costs to customers, particularly in rural areas. Farmers groups and news media[3] highlighted concerns that these changes resulted in difficulties accessing health and emergency care. When services and infrastructure are less accessible in rural communities, it is not only farmers and community members who are affected. Consider this: would you spend a few weeks working on a farm, helping to harvest a crop or muster livestock, and staying in a community with limited options for shopping, entertainment or even patchy mobile reception? Now consider that the work is physically demanding, dirty and probably pays less than a casual job in the city. If you feel disinclined to take up casual farm work, you wouldn't be alone (Foley & Bonyhady, 2020). Not only is it demanding, insecure and low-paid work, it is also in one of Australia's most dangerous industries. This is due to a range of hazards that include farm machinery, chemicals, exposure to the sun and weather, animals, dust and noise.[4]

Now imagine you are a farmer. You have spent months raising your crops or livestock and need short-term help to get your harvest to market so you can pay your bills and purchase inputs for the next crop. Your margins are tight because you compete in global markets where other countries' governments subsidise their farmers, enabling them to offer their produce at lower prices. Australia, in contrast, has among the lowest levels of agricultural subsidies in the Organisation for Economic Cooperation and Development (OECD)[5] with already comparatively low levels of subsidisation slashed during the 1980s and 1990s. If you're lucky, your options for selling your harvest won't be impacted unexpectedly by the actions of federal politicians, such as when, in 2011, live cattle exports were suddenly banned following a media exposé on animal cruelty (*Stock & Land*, 2021), or in 2020 when comments made about the government of China prompted Australia's biggest trading partner to halt imports of many key Australian agricultural commodities (Walker, 2020).

When you combine the difficulties of geographic isolation, long hours of physically demanding work, labour shortages, limited control over costs and income, unpredictable weather and now a changing climate, it is not surprising that farmers report high levels of stress. Research has shown that these factors which affect the physical and mental health of farmers are common both in Australia and internationally (Austin et al., 2018; Yadz et al., 2019). Despite these health challenges, the vast distances that separate Australian farming communities from larger populations mean that, as one group of researchers highlighted in the title of their study into Australian farmers' use of health services, 'We're lucky to have doctors at all' (Hull et al., 2022). After all, health professionals, like seasonal farm workers, can generally find more opportunities and greater amenities by living and working in cities than they can in small rural communities.

How can policymakers address the needs of farming communities effectively without bringing farms closer to cities? One way has been to use migration policies to direct permanent and temporary visa applicants and working holidaymakers to regional areas to fill labour shortages. This has been supported by influential farming industry groups who rely heavily on short-term migrant labour and have for some time lobbied the federal government for a visa tailored to the agriculture sector.[6] In response, the Liberal-National Coalition Government announced the Australian Agriculture Visa Program in the lead-up to the 2022 federal election, however, the election was won by the Australian Labor Party and the new government promptly scrapped the new agriculture visa, opting instead to expand and update the existing Pacific Australia Labour Mobility (PALM) scheme. The PALM scheme aims to address unskilled and semi-skilled labour shortages across several industries and geographic locations. Similarly, governments have tried to address the chronic shortage of health professionals in regional and remote communities by offering a range of skilled visa options to applicants willing to work in regional areas,[7] as well as supporting regional education and placements for trainee health professionals.[8]

The use of migration policies to fill workforce shortages may help farmers and rural communities, but how might it impact the health and wellbeing of migrant workers? Concerns about underpayment and substandard working conditions on Australian farms have been raised by numerous bodies, including researchers, labour unions, and the Fair Work Ombudsman.[9], [10] This is part of a much larger global challenge highlighted by the International Labour Organization, which reported in 2016 that even in high-income countries, migrant farm workers receive low pay for physically demanding work and are unlikely to report exploitation for fear of losing future work (Martin, 2016).

So far, we have considered how small populations in rural, regional and remote areas make it more difficult and less economically viable to provide the same services enjoyed by people in cities and towns. Now let's consider why those places are so sparsely populated. Is it simply a fact of life that farming areas will be less populated?

Population migration

Since the early 1900s, urban populations have been growing faster than total population (Figure 6.1). In Australia, the percentage of the population living in urban areas rose from 60% in 1911 to 90% in 2016.[11] People have migrated from rural to urban areas for many reasons, often in search of better employment, education and services. The historic decline in rural employment opportunities was due at least in part to a reduction in agricultural jobs resulting from farm consolidation and agricultural technologies that improve farming efficiency, thereby reducing the need for human labour. The disappearance of farm jobs has flow-on effects for the surrounding communities. As farm workers migrate to cities in search of work, businesses in rural areas have fewer customers. If the customer base becomes too small, businesses may close or relocate to larger towns. This means fewer services and off-farm jobs available for remaining local populations, and a stronger incentive to move to where the services and opportunities are greater. For small communities, the exodus of people and businesses can become a downward spiral.

For those who do remain, the loss of services can be particularly problematic. The median age of owner-operator farmers in Australia has been steadily increasing, reaching 56 years of

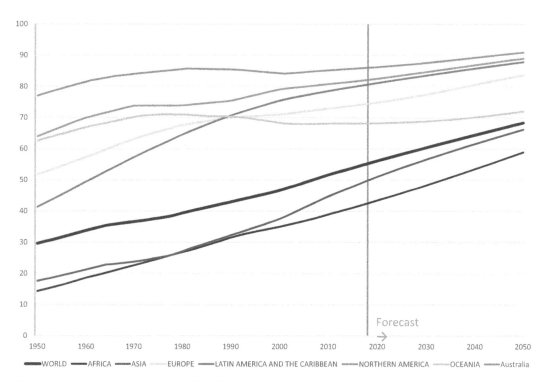

Figure 6.1 Percentage of the population living in urban (versus rural) locations 1950 to 2050
Source: Data from the United Nations Department of Economic and Social Affairs (DESA), World Urbanization Prospects 2018 database.

age at the 2016 census. This makes agriculture the sector with the oldest owner-operators in Australia (Barr & Kancans, 2020). As people age, chronic diseases become more prevalent so the need for health care and other services increases. Declining populations can also mean fewer opportunities to connect with others, undermining the social wellbeing of the community – something which further highlights the criticality of telecommunications infrastructure to support online connection.

What role, if any, has policy played in the rural-to-urban population shift? Agriculture policy in Australia has encouraged farmers to improve efficiency by adopting labour-saving technologies, and to consolidate into fewer and larger farming enterprises to lower costs and increase productivity. This has an obvious impact on farm jobs and rural populations. Yet at the same time, regional development policies have sought to encourage people to live in regional and rural areas, while transport and infrastructure policies have promised to provide those areas with adequate infrastructure and transport links. Why would government policies simultaneously encourage both more and fewer opportunities in agricultural regions?

As with food and nutrition, the policy landscape affecting agriculture and rural communities is broad and complex. Farming communities are impacted by policies spanning the domains of agriculture, infrastructure, transport, environment, education, employment, immigration, trade, social security, land use planning, biosecurity, and more. Since responsibility for these policy domains resides with multiple ministers and government departments, it is common for the policies to have gaps, overlaps and even contradictory objectives. These objectives are often a response to advocacy and lobbying from various interest groups with quite diverse interests.

Spotlight: Policy process

Different interests, different objectives, different policies

Different policy outcomes deliver benefits to some beneficiaries with neutral or even negative impacts for others. Consider these three sets of outcomes, policies and interest groups (Table 6.1).

Table 6.1 Examples of policies meeting different objectives with potential unintended consequences

Policy outcomes	Who benefits	Policy examples	Possible adverse impacts
Increased agricultural efficiency, higher yields, lower costs	Farm owner-operators, commercial farms, agricultural investors, governments (through increased tax revenue)	Delivering Ag2030 (2021); Australia's Tech Future (2018); Rural Research & Development Policy Statement (2012)	Farm jobs lost to technology; environmental impacts of monoculture systems and agri-chemicals; oversupply of foods that dietary guidelines recommend limiting, e.g., red meat, grains, sugar, wine
Support vibrant rural and regional communities with local jobs, education, services and amenities	Rural residents, agricultural workers, local businesses	National Regional, Rural and Remote Tertiary Education Strategy (2019); Planning for Australia's Future Population (2019)	If poorly coordinated, people encouraged to migrate to regions without the jobs and infrastructure to support them, or funds invested in services and infrastructure without the population to use and maintain them

Policy outcomes	Who benefits	Policy examples	Possible adverse impacts
Protect food security and nutrition, promote sustainable food supply	General public, the health system, the environment	Becoming Carbon Neutral by 2030 (MLA, 2020); Climate Change Policy (NFF, 2021); Policy position statement – The Food System, Diet and the Environment (PHAA, 2021)	Policies may be seen as protectionist, discouraging international trade or farm productivity and efficiency; taxpayer funding may be wasted on ineffective environmental initiatives

The primary purpose of commercial enterprise is to maximise total returns to shareholders. This applies to the large-scale industrial farms that now occupy most of Australia's farmland, particularly those that exist as commercial entities owned by investors rather than resident farmers. In agriculture, economic returns are maximised by specialising in commodities that can be produced efficiently and sold for a reasonable price, and by investing in valuable assets such as prime farmland and water rights. The profit motive stands in contrast to, and often in conflict with, other outcomes that support public health such as supplying a diversity of fresh healthy foods at a reasonable price to consumers, selecting crop and livestock varieties that prioritise nutritional traits over some others like fast growth, and enhancing rather than degrading natural ecosystems. Decades of policies that encouraged farm consolidation, industrialisation, capital investments by non-farmer investors, and specialisation in highly profitable commodities for export markets have contributed to unintended consequences beyond the reduction of agriculture and non-agriculture jobs in rural areas. They have also contributed to an agri-food system that is now recognised as a major contributor to climate change, biodiversity loss, water depletion and pollution. We turn to this next.

Climate

Indigenous perspective

Is it possible to feed populations sustainably from Australian soils, often described as ancient and fragile?

Before the British colonisers arrived in 1788, the peoples of the hundreds of Aboriginal and Torres Strait Islander nations that occupied the land managed it sustainably for thousands of generations. The practices used to care for Country were carefully refined over at least 70,000 years. During this time, the people and country adapted to massive changes in temperature and sea level, and the extinction of megafauna species.

Carefully controlled burning, animal husbandry, cropping and tool technologies are among the agricultural practices detailed in the works of historian Adjunct Professor Bill Gammage, Bunurong writer and farmer Professor Bruce Pascoe, scientist Professor Tim Flannery and others. Sustainability is a defining feature of the life, culture and land management practices of Australia's First Peoples. As Pascoe explains: 'Aboriginal people are born of the earth and individuals within the clan had responsibilities for particular streams, grasslands, trees, crops, animals and even seasons. The life of the clan was devoted to continuance' (2016, p. 145).

When we discussed the sources of stress for farmers, we considered how lack of control over weather and climate are among the many challenges farmers face. This is because farming is critically dependent upon environmental conditions and can be (and increasingly is) devastated by extreme weather events such as floods and prolonged droughts. According to the International Panel on Climate Change, current climate trends are likely to make future conditions far more challenging for farmers in Australia and around the world (IPCC, 2019). The climate certainly impacts agriculture, but this relationship is not one-way. Industrialised agricultural practices have been associated with carbon dioxide emissions through the use of fossil fuels to power farm machinery and to transport inputs and produce across global supply chains. The carbon from fossil fuels has been locked away under the Earth's surface since the Carboniferous Age, when the Earth was much hotter than it is today. The release of this carbon is adding to the blanket of greenhouse gases that are returning our climate to warmer conditions. In addition, carbon is released from soil and vegetation by ploughing and burning. This organic matter, if allowed to decompose biologically, would improve the health and water-holding capacity of soil by building soil carbon. However, when released as carbon dioxide, it adds to the greenhouse gases causing global heating, while also depleting soil and contributing to erosion. Policies of successive Australian governments, our global trading partners and international agencies, like the World Trade Organization and Food and Agriculture Organization (FAO), have encouraged the adoption of industrial agriculture and global trade of agricultural products for decades without adequately mitigating the impacts of greenhouse gas emissions produced through industrialised farming practices and fossil fuel-reliant transport. More recently, the UN Environment Programme (UNEP) has called for transformation of agri-food systems to address their negative impacts on planetary health and ensure food production can continue sustainably into the future.

Global context: Repurposing agricultural support

In 2021, a major report by the UN Environment Programme (UNEP), UN Development Programme (UNDP) and the Food and Agriculture Organization (FAO) called for an overhaul of government subsidies and supports of the agriculture sector. The report found that most of the existing supports 'distort food prices, hurt people's health, and degrade the environment'. This is a major concern since the value of global agricultural supports was forecast to reach USD1.8 trillion by 2030. But it also represents an enormous opportunity.

Existing subsidies harm human and planetary health by promoting chemical use and emissions-intensive farming sectors. They also predominantly support large-scale agriculture while neglecting smallholder farmers. Small farms are, on average, more productive per hectare under cultivation and provide nutrition and livelihoods for many of the world's most disadvantaged people. The report calls for governments to redirect subsidies towards supporting agricultural practices that are healthy, sustainable and equitable. This includes investing in public infrastructure and services such as agricultural research and development.

The full report is available at: www.unep.org/resources/repurposing-agricultural-support-transform-food-systems

While Australia provides relatively little public subsidisation of ongoing agricultural activities, the government is generally responsive when the sector experiences extreme climate events, such as drought or flood. For example, low-interest loans and financial counselling are available to drought affected farmers and farming families experiencing hardship can access a Farm Household Allowance for up to four years.[12] The provision of emergency support appears to contradict the neoliberal ideology of small government and free markets. Under neoliberal ideology, agricultural enterprises would be expected to pay for insurance, or self-insure to cover the costs of any natural disasters. Why would governments make exceptions for farmers during a drought but not subsidise them to supply the ongoing dietary needs of Australians? Part of the reason seems to be strong public sentiment in support of farmers. Past research tells us that farming and family farms form part of the Australian cultural identity, and images of farmers in crisis elicit strong public sympathy (Botterill, 2016; Cullerton et al., 2022). Public opinion can have a strong influence over government policy, even when it runs counter to the governing party's ideological stance (Cullerton et al., 2016).

Why, then, if more than four out of five Australians want stronger government action on climate change (Colvin & Jotzo, 2021), have successive Australian governments been slow to adopt policies that address greenhouse gas emissions from the agriculture sector? One possible reason is the low public awareness of the agriculture sector's contribution to climate change. A recent study found that although food systems are known to be responsible for a third of global greenhouse gas emissions, Australian media coverage of climate change mentioned food systems only 5% of the time. In fact, they were more likely to mention the impact climate change is having on food systems, than the effects food systems have on the climate (Atkinson et al., 2022).

Spotlight: Advocacy action

Net zero by 2050

With a third of greenhouse gas emissions coming from the food and agriculture sector, you would think reducing agriculture emissions would be an important target for climate policy. However, Australian Governments have attracted criticism for lacking ambition on climate action, ranking last for climate policy in the Climate Change Performance Index in 2021 and very poor overall for climate policy and performance for 2022 and 2023.

In 2020, the National Farmers Federation (NFF), Australia's peak body representing farmers, called on the Liberal-National Coalition Government to adopt the target of net zero carbon emissions by 2050 across the entire economy, including agriculture. Despite the NFF historically having considerable sway over government policies, the government proved slow to take up this challenge. Initially, then Agriculture Minister David Littleproud rejected the NFF's proposal. This is despite the agriculture sector already having made significant progress on emissions reduction and the red meat sector represented by Meat and Livestock Australia (MLA), traditionally seen as one of the most emissions-intensive sectors, having already adopted a more ambitious target of net zero by 2030.

So aware are Australian farmers of the impacts of climate change that the sector has already made substantial progress on innovations to reduce its impact and adapt to locked-in changes, such as methane-reducing additives to livestock feed and climate-smart crop and livestock breeds. Since 2015, farmers have also lobbied governments to adopt strong economy-wide climate policies through the advocacy group Farmers For Climate Action. Farmers have a vested interest in strong climate policy for several reasons. First, they are directly impacted by climate change through more severe droughts, floods, fires and pests. Second, the marketability of Australia's agricultural products is impacted while Australia lacks credible climate policies. Third, there are opportunities for farmers and farming communities to benefit from good climate policy. These range from incentives to protect habitat and sequester carbon, to public investment in sustainable agriculture research, through to additional income from supplying surplus renewable energy to the electricity grid.

It was more than a year after the NFF urged the federal Liberal-National Coalition Government to set a net zero 2050 target that it eventually unveiled its policy in late 2021. However, it was the subsequent federal Labor Government that finally legislated the target of net zero by 2050 in its Climate Change Bill 2022, the following year.

Let's finish

We have explored how politics and policy affect health in the context of food systems and agriculture. By now you will be aware of several themes that permeate the topic. First, the links between food and agricultural systems and health are well established, and significant. Food system drivers of unhealthy diets – especially the production, marketing, and consumption of ultra-processed food – are also key drivers of nutrition-related disease. Unsustainable agricultural practices are impacting planetary health and climate stability, and the choices farmers make about what to produce – based on policy that promotes production of cash crops for export markets and for use in ultra-processed foods – also impact the diversity and healthy nature of the foods available to consumers. Second, policymaking in food systems is complex. Achieving better health outcomes requires coherent and coordinated policy implementation across a broad range of policy domains. Further, it must respond to the needs of many different interest groups, often with competing interests. This leads to the third issue.

There is considerable inequity in different groups' power to influence policy, and consequently, in the distribution of benefits and harms. Population health depends on food systems that are both effective and equitable. We have seen how the food industry uses a range of practices to ensure policies reflect their interests. Yet while industry profits, the wider population is experiencing rising rates of both diet-related diseases and food insecurity, along with environmental and climate impacts. Food is a political matter. Whether food systems change depends on who gains or loses from the changes. How can we transition a country and its decision-makers into thinking about the long-term impacts of policy decisions around food and farming? How can we balance the significant power of the food industry and elevate the voices of those affected by food insecurity and diet-related disease? And if we could agree on policy objectives that support healthier outcomes, how can we transform systems that span so many different domains?

Summary

The ways our food is produced impacts not only the nutrition it provides but also planetary health. Therefore significant benefits can accrue from improving our food environments. This includes not only health and environmental benefits but also financial benefits. However, food is a political matter. Whether food systems change depends on who gains or loses from the changes.

After studying this chapter, you should now be able to:

- Understand how governments influence food systems and planetary health.
- Identify key actors in Australian food policy, their interests, and the ways they influence policy agendas and outcomes.

- Assess the health impacts of different policy priorities for food and nutrition.
- Understand the major challenges and opportunities for farmers.
- Compare the breadth of policy domains that impact farming communities.
- Identify the interactions between food production, the environment and climate, and the political influences on these relationships.

Tutorial exercises

1   Each element of the food system has both benefits and costs associated with people (farmers, neighbours, consumers), the environment, and the economy. In groups, identify the positive and/or negative impacts to the environment, people and the economy for each part of the food system.
2   Policy actions in one part of the food system have consequences for other parts of the system. Can you identify a policy designed to address one aspect of the food system that might have consequences in another part?
3   Choose a food system problem to address. Describe the impact of the problem on public health, society and/or ecosystems. Identify the factors that contribute to the problem and choose one of these where you would like to lobby to change. Who could be allies who could lobby with you? Who would oppose this change and how could they be overcome?
4   To gain a better understanding of transnational food and beverage companies and how they operate, identify the largest (by income) five transnational food or beverage organisations. What is their annual income? How wide is their product range? How many countries do they operate in? Are they publicly listed companies or privately owned?

Notes

1 See WHO (2017).
2 For a discussion of concepts and definitions of regional and rural compared to urban and metropolitan areas in Australia, see Dadpour and Law (2022).
3 See, for example, Gregory (2005) and Bowyer et al. (2020).
4 See agriculture industry information at Safe Work Australia, available at: https://www.safeworkaustralia.gov.au/safety-topic/industry-and-business/agriculture
5 See OECD data on agricultural support for Australia, available at: https://data.oecd.org/agrpolicy/agricultural-support.htm
6 See the National Farmers Federation issues statement on a dedicated agriculture visa on their website, available at: https://nff.org.au/key-issue/dedicated-agriculture-visa/
7 For more information on skilled visa options, see the Australian Government Department of Home Affairs website, available at: https://immi.homeaffairs.gov.au/visas/getting-a-visa/visa-finder
8 For an analysis of the effectiveness of policies to regionalise health professional training, see Carson, McGrail and Sahay (2022).
9 Listen to Australian Council of Trade Unions President Michele O'Neill on ABC radio: 'ACTU warns new Ag visa risks foreign workers being treated like property', 11 November 2021, available at: https://www.abc.net.au/radionational/programs/breakfast/actu-warns-new-ag-visa-risks-foreign-workers-exploitation/13626230
10 See media releases at the Australian Fair Work Ombudsman's website, including 'FWO fines farm employers more than $78,000', 9 December 2022, available at: https://www.fairwork.gov.au/newsroom/media-releases/2022-media-releases/december-2022/20221209-agriculture-inspections-december-2022-media-release
11 Census data is published on the Australian Bureau of Statistics website, available at: www.abs.gov.au
12 For current government assistance for farmers, see the Department of Agriculture, Fisheries and Forestry website, available at: www.agriculture.gov.au

Further reading

Chan, G. (2021). *Why you should give a f*ck about farming*. Melbourne, Victoria: Vintage Books.

FAO, IFAD, UNICEF, WFP & WHO. (2022). *The state of food security and nutrition in the world, 2022*. Rome: FAO.

Farmers for Climate Action. Available at: www.farmersforclimateaction.org.au

Holmes, T.*et al.* (2012). *The common cause handbook*. London: Public Interest Research Centre.

Mann, A. (2021). *Food in a changing climate*. Bingley: Emerald Publishing Limited.

Swinburn, B.*et al.* (2019). The global syndemic of obesity, undernutrition, and climate change: The Lancet Commission report. *The Lancet*, 393(10173), 791–846.

WHO. (2017). *Tackling NCDs: 'Best Buys' and Other Recommended Interventions for the Prevention and Control of Noncommunicable Diseases*. Geneva: WHO.

Willett, W.*et al.* (2019). Food in the Anthropocene: The EAT–Lancet Commission on healthy diets from sustainable food systems. *The Lancet*, 393(10170), 447–492.

References

Atkinson, N., Ferguson, M., Russell, C., & Cullerton, K. (2022). Are the impacts of food systems on climate change being reported by the media? An Australian media analysis. *Public Health Nutrition*, 27, 1–9.

Austin, E. K.et al. (2018). Drought-related stress among farmers: Findings from the Australian Rural Mental Health Study. *The Medical Journal of Australia*, 209(4): 159–165.

Barr, N., & Kancans, R. (2020). Trends in the Australian Agricultural Workforce: What can data from the Census of Population and Housing tell us about changes in agricultural employment? ABARES Research Report 20.19. Canberra: ABARES.

Booth, S., & Pollard, C. M. (2020). Food insecurity, food crimes and structural violence: An Australian perspective. *Australian and New Zealand Journal of Public Health*, 44, 87–88.

Botterill, L. C. (2016). Agricultural policy in Australia: Deregulation, bipartisanship and agrarian senti-ment. *Australian Journal of Political Science*, 51(4), 667–682.

Bowyer, D., Jones, G., Bowrey, G., & Smark, C. (2020). Survival of the fittest? Challenges to regional aviation and regional communities from the privatisation of Australia's airports. *Australasian Journal of Regional Studies*, 26(1), 1–28.

Branca, F.et al. (2019). Transforming the food system to fight non-communicable diseases. *BMJ*, 364.

Brimblecombe, J.et al. (2020). Effect of restricted retail merchandising of discretionary food and beverages on population diet: A pragmatic randomised controlled trial. *The Lancet Planetary Health*, 4(10), e463–e473.

Caraher, M., & Furey, S. (2018). Growth of food banks in the UK (and Europe): Leftover food for left-over people. In *The economics of emergency food aid provision*. Cham: Palgrave Pivot.

Carey, R.et al. (2016). Opportunities and challenges in developing a whole-of-government national food and nutrition policy: Lessons from Australia's National Food Plan. *Public Health Nutrition*, 19(1), 3–14.

Carson, D. B., McGrail, M., & Sahay, A. (2022). Regionalisation and general practitioner and nurse workforce development in regional northern Australia: Insights from 30 years of census migration data. *Journal of Rural Studies*, 91, 98–107.

Cicchini, S., Lee, A., & Cullerton, K. (2021). Who votes for public health? An analysis of Australian politicians' parliamentary voting behaviour. *Public Health Research and Practice*, 31(3), 30342014.

Cohen, J. E.*et al.* (2000). Political ideology and tobacco control. *Tobacco Control*, 9(3), 263–267.

Colvin, R., & Jotzo, F. (2021). If 80% of Australians care about climate action, why don't they vote like it? *The Conversation*, 25 March 2021.

Crippa, M.*et al.* (2021). Food systems are responsible for a third of global anthropogenic GHG emissions. *Nature Food*, 2(3), 198–209.

Crosland, P.*et al.* (2019). The economic cost of preventable disease in Australia: A systematic review of estimates and methods. *Australian and New Zealand Journal of Public Health*, 43, 484–495.

Cullerton, K., Donnet, T., Lee, A.*et al.* (2016). Playing the policy game: A review of the barriers to and enablers of nutrition policy change. *Public Health Nutrition*, 19(14), 2643–2653.

Cullerton, K., Patay, D., Waller, M.*et al.* (2022). Competing public narratives in nutrition policy: Insights into the ideational barriers of public support for regulatory nutrition measures. *Health Research Policy and Systems*, 20, 86.

Dadpour, R., & Law, L. (2022). Understanding the 'region' in COVID-19-induced regional migration: Mapping Cairns across classification systems. *Australian Geographer*, 53(4), 425–443.

FAO, IFAD, UNICEF, WFP, & WHO. (2021). *The state of food security and nutrition in the world, 2021: Transforming food systems for food security, improved nutrition and affordable healthy diets for all.* Rome: FAO.

FAO, IFAD, UNICEF, WFP, & WHO. (2022). *The state of food security and nutrition in the world, 2022.* Rome: FAO.

Foley, M., & Bonyhady, N. (2020). Farm labour shortage risks food price spike as Aussies shun harvest jobs. *The Sydney Morning Herald*, 11 August.

Friedman, M. (1962). *Capitalism and freedom.* Chicago: University of Chicago Press.

Gregory, G. (2005). Health, Telstra and the future: A rural perspective. *Impact*, (Spring), 17–19.

Holmes, T.*et al.* (2012). *The common cause handbook.* London: Public Interest Research Centre.

Hull, M. J.*et al.* (2022). "We're lucky to have doctors at all": A qualitative exploration of Australian farmers' barriers and facilitators to health-related help-seeking. *International Journal of Environmental Research and Public Health*, 19(17), 11075.

IFPRI. (2021). *2021 Global food policy report: Transforming food systems after COVID-19.* Washington, DC: International Food Policy Research Institute.

IPCC. (2019). *Climate change and land: An IPCC special report on climate change, desertification, land degradation, sustainable land management, food security, and greenhouse gas fluxes in terrestrial ecosystems.* Geneva: IPCC.

IPES-Food. (2016). From uniformity to diversity: A paradigm shift from industrial agriculture to diversified agroecological systems. International Panel of Experts on Sustainable Food Systems. Available at: www.ipes-food.org/_img/upload/files/UniformityTo…

James, S. (2014). Protecting Sydney's peri-urban agriculture: Moving beyond a housing/farming dichotomy . *Geographical Research*, 52(4), 377–386.

Martin, P. L. (2016). *Migrant workers in commercial agriculture.* Geneva: International Labour Organization.

McMichael, P. (2004). *Development and social change: A global perspective.* 3rd edn. Thousand Oaks, CA: Pine Forge Press.

MLA. (2020). Becoming carbon neutral by 2030. Meat & Livestock Australia. Available at: https://www.mla.com.au/globalassets/mla-corporate/research-and-development/documents/cn30-information-sheet-final.pdf

Nestle, M. (2002). *Food politics: How the food industry influences nutrition and health.* Berkeley, CA: University of California Press.

Nestle, M. (2013). *Eat drink vote: An illustrated guide to food politics.* New York: Rodale.

NFF. (2021). Climate change policy. National Farmers Federation. Available at: https://nff.org.au/wp-content/uploads/2021/03/NFF_Factsheet_Climate-Change-Policy_2021A-1.pdf

NHMRC. (2013). Australian dietary guidelines-Providing the scientific evidence for healthier Australian diets. Canberra: NHMRC.

Pascoe, B. (2016). *Dark emu black seeds: Agriculture or accident?*Broome, Western Australia: Magabala Books.

PHAA (Public Health Association of Australia). (2021). The food system: Diet and the environment – Policy position statement. Available at: https://www.phaa.net.au/documents/item/5253 (accessed 21 November 2022).

Stock & Land (2021). Decade since live-export ban. *Stock & Land*, 10 June.

UNEP. (2021). *UNEP Food Waste Index report 2021.* Nairobi: United Nations Environment Programme.

Walker, T. (2020). Timeline of a broken relationship: How China and Australia went from chilly to barely speaking. *The Conversation*, 9 December 2020.

WHO. (2017). *Tackling NCDs: 'Best buys' and other recommended interventions for the prevention and control of noncommunicable diseases.* Geneva: World Health Organization.

WHO. (2022). *World health statistics, 2022: Monitoring health for the SDGs, Sustainable Development Goals.* Geneva: World Health Organization.

Yazd, S. D., Wheeler, S. A., & Zuo, A. (2019). Key risk factors affecting farmers' mental health: A systematic review. *International Journal of Environmental Research and Public Health*, 16(23): 4849.

7 Waste and Water

Nina Lansbury and Marguerite C. Sendall

The General Assembly,

1. Recognizes the right to safe and clean drinking water and sanitation as a human right that is essential for the full enjoyment of life and all human rights.

2. Calls upon States and international organizations to provide financial resources, capacity-building and technology transfer, through international assistance and cooperation, in particular to developing countries, in order to scale up efforts to provide safe, clean, accessible and affordable drinking water and sanitation for all.

(The human right to water and sanitation (A/RES/64/292), United Nations (2010)).

Learning objectives

After studying this chapter, you should be able to:

1 Understand household waste production and approaches to recycling, reusing and revaluing household waste.
2 Critique approaches to managing commercial waste including landfill and the circular economy from a planetary perspective.
3 Critically analyse the ethics and sustainability of the fast and slow fashion industry and the implications for health.
4 Recognise the challenges of delivering safe and acceptable drinking water and wastewater treatment now and in a climate-affected future.
5 Evaluate aspects of essential service of water and wastewater delivery affected by political decisions.
6 Synthesise features of water and wastewater management beyond technological solutions to include social, financial and cultural aspects.

Snapshot

A safe glass of drinking water in Australia in 2023

In 2015, Australia pledged to attain the UN Sustainable Development Goals (SDGs) by 2030, including SDG6 to 'Ensure availability and sustainable management of water and sanitation for all'. However, when detailing the country's progress in their mandated reporting to the UN on SDG status (DFAT, 2018), the Government noted that not all Australians had the same access to safe and reliable drinking water. They stated:

DOI: 10.4324/9781003315490-12

Rural and remote communities may not have the same level of access to water and sanitation services as urban centres. This is particularly the case for remote Aboriginal and Torres Strait Islander communities and can have important flow on effects to health outcomes.

(DFAT, 2018, p. 50)

More recently, a report was released regarding the drinking water of the regional town of Walgett in New South Wales, where almost half the population are Aboriginal people. The report detailed how the town was 'without reliable, safe or acceptable drinking water' due to 'systematic water mismanagement which, exacerbated by both drought and flood, has rendered surface water supplies unreliable and produced high levels of water insecurity for Walgett residents' (Earle et al, 2023, p, 2). Walgett's drinking water contains high concentrations of sodium that impact chronic conditions including hypertension and kidney disease (Earle et al, 2023).

Providing context to this scenario is another report, which found tap water in over 500 remote Indigenous communities was not regularly tested and often not safe to drink. The supply was contaminated microbially (through bacteria and viruses) and chemically through both naturally occurring levels of uranium, arsenic, fluoride and nitrates, as well as through industrial pollution. The issues presented in the Snapshot above pose risks to human health and ecological health.

Let's begin

This chapter will explore contemporary, futuristic and often double-barrelled issues related to waste and water as they affect human health. The first half of this chapter is about waste. It begins with the concept of consumption and the production of household waste and considers the infrastructure required to manage recycling of household waste. Recently, China has imposed sanctions on the importation of waste, and the impact of this ban on Australia is explored. This section takes a close look at two of the 'big issues' of waste: single-use plastic and batteries. It presents issues and ideas associated with open defecation and the humble toilet. Commercial waste from a political and planetary perspective is explored. Landfill and the circular economy are discussed in the context of healthcare before considering waste management strategies adopted in the global context. Next, the role of government, industry and other stakeholders and innovative strategies in waste management are explored. In particular, nickel mining and associated cultural concerns as well as nuclear energy are discussed. The last section of the chapter on waste introduces the fast and slow fashion industry, posing queries on ethical production and supply chains, consumerism, consumer demand and consumer activism. The second half of this chapter is about water. You will learn how water is essential to human existence and linked to human health, from the basic ability for the human body to stay hydrated and alive to the health impacts from contaminated water. Political determinants of health are explained throughout this chapter regarding the challenge of maintaining and providing safe and acceptable ('potable and palatable') drinking water and of adequately and safely managing wastewater (sewage). This will include a reflection on the range of water-related 'neglected tropical diseases' that affect millions of people who live in low-income countries. Funding and efforts to ensure safe drinking water and sewage management appear to be neglected or deprioritised due to reasons other than the high burden of disease that these cause; it could well be considered that poverty creates an invisibility from political priorities. Both halves of this chapter close with opportunities for sustainable management options that value the resources of so-called waste and of precious water.

Waste: The health impacts of the politics of waste and waste policy

Households

Underpinning the concept of waste and waste management is consumption. Over-consumption is a global phenomenon that emerged after the industrial revolution, and it has profited through modern events such as wars. It is fuelled by the technological age and our desire for new 'things'. Simply put, we as humans like accumulating 'stuff', sometimes needfully but often needlessly. Over-consumption is political, for example, what is the role of business, the government or stock markets? There are ethical reactions, such as anti-consumerism and a growing degrowth movement which illustrate reactions and emerging positive actions. From a social perspective, who do sustainable options impact, and how? With the highest footprint in the G20 countries, Australian households produce more than 2 million tonnes of hard and soft plastic per annum. This footprint has implications for the UN Sustainable Development Goal (SDG) 12: Responsible consumption and production (United Nations, 2015a). Being cautious not to blame individuals, families and households, there are conscious steps which can be taken to reduce over-consumption. Note: Soon there will be more plastic in the oceans than fish. Simply put, we need to use less plastic. Looking forward, new infrastructure is needed to manage the recycling of more and more plastic waste and at the same time, consider risks to human and planetary health. Cook, Velis and Cottom (2022) conducted a rapid review of the potential risks of plastic packaging waste collected and separated for recycling. The findings indicate the process least likely to impact the environment is mechanical reprocessing and the best option for developing countries to implement. Chemical recycling processes are immature, it is difficult to assess their real-world impacts on human health and the environment and at present, these are not helpful to the circular economy in the Global South. The authors suggest flexible, multi-material and multi-layer products suited to mechanical recycling should be targeted for circular economy activity but suggest barriers to shifting the dominant resource recovery mode to other emerging recovery approaches. We'll revisit the circular economy later in this chapter.

Broadly speaking, we can say Australians are wasteful per person (including food waste discussed in Chapter 6: Food and farming) but somewhat good at collecting and sorting recyclable waste. However, the Australian waste management business is not good at managing our recyclable waste; that is, they do not buy our recyclable plastic, paper and cardboard so we sell much of it to China. In 2018, China enforced sanctions on the importation of foreign waste because it was heavily contaminated, costly to clean and they had invested in more sophisticated recycling systems. At that time, China accepted about 30%, or more than 600,000 tonnes, of Australia's recyclable waste. Australia no longer meets China's requirements for importation of recyclable waste. Essentially, China's waste pipeline has dried up. Since the ban by China, Australia has been left with a dilemma. Mountains of recyclable waste is now bound for landfill which compounds an existing problem and has significant implications for human and planetary health. There has been a significant financial shift in the recycling market. For example, Australians purchase white glass as packaging for food stuffs and put it in the recycling bin. Most of this white glass is sent to landfill because there is no profit margin for glass recycling. Similarly, cardboard used to sell for $120 per tonne and now sells for $60 per tonne. So, should Australia find new markets for its waste? Or should/could Australia seize this as an opportunity to reconsider its 'waste' as a valuable resource?

Single-use plastics are part of our daily and household lives – known as mundane consumption – to carry our groceries, collect our dry cleaning, drink our bottled water and deliver our takeaway dinner. Australians use more than 1 million tonnes of takeaway plastic containers every year but only 16% of these containers are recovered for recycling or reuse. The national target for recovery is 70%, but experts suggest until the industry is regulated, this is unlikely to be achieved and any real impact on planetary, and ultimately human health will be delayed. Broadly speaking, this has consequences for UN SDG12. Some councils in Australia have taken a proactive approach. Hobart City Council is a good example: one decade ago, the Council implemented a waste management strategy to phase out plastic and phase in compostable takeaway food containers at the point of sale at festivals and community events. The Council manages this strategy akin to food inspections through regular checks and fines. Despite varying costs to businesses, many have already switched to compostable takeaway food containers, including more than 300 stalls at Salamanca markets. The Council mandates the eco-friendly packaging materials should be compostable (that is, break down to organic matter) but some compostable products can still contain microplastics. For example, the inside of disposable coffee cups are plastic. Hobart Council is clear about the need for improved labelling because the recycling symbol is commonly misunderstood. Waste management communication experts recommend a simple labelling system, like a 'traffic light system' for the front of food packages or household garbage bins that could be more easily understood.

Household batteries are also part of our daily and household lives. Think about your battery-powered day. From the time you get out of bed until you go back to bed, how many battery-powered products do you use? From the battery in your alarm clock, toothbrush, TV and air conditioning remote controls, children's toys, power tools, devices and car or e-bikes. How many of these batteries do you recharge or recycle? Australians use approximately 150 million batteries annually. This number is expected to increase as Australians use more batteries, particularly for powering technology. By 2050, the World Bank expects the global demand for batteries will grow by 500%. This alone is a strong argument for recycling batteries and to minimise the impact on our planet's health. Other arguments for recycling batteries include a short supply of manufacturing materials and reducing environmental impact by limiting the amount of corrosive and toxic materials which end up in landfill. In recently published research, Takefuji (2022) compares lithium batteries used in smartphones to asbestos. Asbestos was hailed as a dream material when it was invented because it was, among other things, very accessible and available. The human health problems associated with asbestos are now well documented. While lithium batteries do not contain hazardous substances, when heated, they produce toxic gases and, if they are damaged, may cause a fire or explosion hazard, particularly at the end of their life. The author presents findings of a members survey conducted by the Environmental Services Association, UK, which found 145 of 670 fires recorded in 2019–2020 were attributed directly to lithium batteries. According to the UK Consumer Product Safety Commission's Status Report on High Energy Density Batteries Project (2018), between January 2012 and July 2017, approximately 25,000 overheating or fire incidents involved at least 400 types of lithium battery-powered products. Despite these findings, lithium batteries have been greenwashed. What do you understand by the concept of 'green washing'? What other products have been greenwashed and mislead the consumer?

Limelight

Have you heard about the about the giant 'fatberg' in the London sewer system? A fatberg is a huge coagulation of waste products, for example, nappies, wet wipes, condoms and a whole bunch of other stuff, which end up in our town and city sewage systems. The fatberg in

London's sewage system is one of biggest known – it weighs about 130 tonnes – that's more than a blue whale, a Boeing 757-200 or a house. The London Fatberg snowballed out of control because the sewer system in London is not well mapped. London isn't the only city which has a fatberg problem. Here is some information about a campaign in the Australian Capital Territory: https://www.iconwater.com.au/My-Home/free-the-poo.aspx. This public information campaign seeks to educate the public about what can be flushed down a toilet to prevent fatberg potential – especially period care products and baby wipes. There are lots of fatbergs around the world but most of them are the size of a tennis or football. Fatbergs start with a small blockage, snowball into much bigger blockages and need to be manually and mechanically broken up. Remember, only the three PPPs (pee, poo, and paper) can go down the sink and the toilet!

There are clear links between waste and water – water is essential for human life and waste is a consequence of living. Waste impacts water in many ways, for example, the role of water in the disposal of human waste. And, if contaminated, it can have severe health consequences as discussed later. In some parts of the world, the disposal of human waste has been an ongoing health issue. Many years ago, cities such as London, Paris, New York and Mumbai built large and intricate underground systems to deal with sewage. But human defaecation has not always been managed in ways which protect human health. History books tell us about the spread of cholera and typhoid from poor sanitation. Indeed, Florence Nightingale discovered that British soldiers fighting in the Crimea in 1853–1856 were more likely to die because of poor sanitation than from being shot. Open defecation, or where people defecate outside (*in the open*) rather than in a toilet, is still a problem especially in large cities in countries like India and many other low-income and highly populated countries. There are many issues associated with open defecation, including a lack of toilets and a lack of functioning toilets. Globally, about 200 million toilets are required to manage open defecation. Alas, it is not as simple as procuring funding and starting production. The big question is: *What is the best toilet?*

Let's think

Let's rethink the humble toilet. Most of us have one, maybe two, and we all use them once a day. But do our toilets align with today's sustainable and environmentally friendly expectations? Have they kept up with modernity? Are they fit for purpose in contextualised human and planetary health paradigms? Over time, plumbed, flushing, water-based toilet design has not kept up with contemporary human health and environmental demands. Composting toilets have become popular in houseboats and vans in regions such as Scandinavia. Sweden has designed a new toilet which maximises the value and reduces the smell of human excreta by separating urine (full of important resources such as nitrite and urea) and faeces (also a useful resource for soil nutrients, if managed well). Experts suggest the perfect toilet doesn't have a sewage system, but standalone toilets need lots of water which is problematic in an increasingly water-depleted world. Other options include toilets that use a membrane or bacteria to produce, for example, fertiliser. The Dutch and Chinese used these sort of toilets hundreds of years ago but today, there are issues with replacing membranes and managing bacteria.

Industry

The idea of a 'circular economy' emerged in the 1970s in a bid to decrease the problem of waste products piling up in refuse centres and landfill sites around the world. Think back to the waste produced from single-use plastic and batteries. The circular economy has been likened to other social movements on issues, such as pollution and waste, linked to climate change. These movements, underpinned by concerns for human and planetary health, share similar traits, such as a clear vision with correlated and identifying language, a strong social responsibility and value and loud advocacy for environmental justice. Syms, Taylor-Robinson and Trovato (2023) suggest the circular economy (that is, being much more thoughtful about how resources are managed) should be adopted by healthcare settings. Circular medicine is critical now because hospitals produce significant quantities of medical and other waste, including unused products. Ironically, very little is reused or recycled in a sustainable way for human and planetary health. These movements are ideologically, philosophically and possibly economically driven, and do not yet offer practical options to turn vision into reality. From a pragmatic perspective, Australia's health sector should commit itself nationally to net zero carbon emissions by 2040, in line with the National Health Service in the UK, preferably with the states and territories responsible for implementing evidence-based interventions (Vardoulakis, 2021). Most importantly, there should be operational accountability. In particular, the healthcare sector broadly has imperatives to meet the SDG 12 targets.

As highlighted in the Limelight box, China has recently sanctioned the import of foreign waste from Australia. One option to address this waste management issue might be to find new markets such as Malaysia, Thailand, India and Indonesia. This approach would be a quick fix and avoid dealing with the heart of the problem. However, the Waste Manage Net and Resource Recovery Association of Australia proposes Australia should re-think its values about waste and waste management from a global perspective by implementing strategies to minimise and manage waste, not just shift waste management offshore. The Association suggests one strategy is to rethink purchasing. This could be regulated at a national level and implemented at state level whereby governments would be accountable for thoughtful requisition. For example, purchasing sand for road construction made from recycled glass. This would drive demand and provide incentives for Australian businesses to develop and build enhanced remanufacturing capacity. However, it requires political will by consumers, industry and politicians including local, state and federal ministers responsible for Waste Education and Environmental Management portfolios. This shift, if enacted, would see Australia catch up, at least in some part, to the EU policy which mandates recycling and benefit the planet's health. Globally, there is a lot of interest in the circular economy, the idea that 'what you make, you take back'. Ironically, China may have inadvertently pushed Australia along this pathway.

Global context

Since the 1990s, Germany has adopted a different attitude to waste management: waste cannot just be dumped; it has to be treated or recycled. More recently, European countries like Sweden have adopted an environmental policy approach called the Extended Producer Responsibility (EPR). The EPR extends the producer's responsibility to the post-consumer stage of a product's life cycle. It shifts responsibility away from councils and users to producers and incentivises producers to design environmentally friendly products. You can find out more information about the EPR from the Organisation for Economic Co-operation and

Development. Here is the link:https://www.oecd.org/environment/extended-producer-resp
onsibility.htm. The EPR has changed the political landscape and appetite in Europe, and
more widely, by putting pressure on producers to actively transition to become better
environmental citizens. In Hong Kong (population 7.413 million, landmass 1,106 square
kilometres), human consumption is high and abundant waste is pumped into one of the
world's busiest harbours, Victoria Harbour, turning it into a smelly sewage dump. This has
immediate and long-term consequences for human health including outbreaks of waterborne
disease and planetary health such as environmental degradation. In 2015, the Hong Kong
government introduced a novel bio-remedial approach, the Harbour Area Treatment Scheme
(HATS). Among other strategies, HATS used oysters, which filter water and reproduce
swiftly, to populate and build a reef to clean up the harbour. Here is more information about
HATS: https://www.epd.gov.hk/epd/english/environmentinhk/water/cleanharbour/home.html
Over the last 8 years, HATS has improved the water quality and the marine environment, has
decreased the public health risk and contributed to economic productivity through ongoing
tourism in this iconic harbour.

Globally, waste and waste management systems are managed in a diversity of ways and have
improved over time. A landmark book in the modern environmental movement, *Silent Spring*
was published by Carson in 1962. It revealed the effect of pesticides on the natural environment, the risk to human health and forced new policies for air and water protection, and in
turn, human and planetary health. Until the 1970s, Australia's foremost waste management
strategy was to locate landfill sites far away from most of the population as possible. This
approach largely absolved waste management companies of responsibility for land, water and
air contamination. Do you think this approach was ethical – that is, was it doing good *and*
doing no harm? Consider the health, social and environmental impacts on those closer to and
further away from landfill sites. It is a similar case with mine sites. Many mines are located
near settlements whose residents who hold little power in comparison to the mining
companies.

Spotlight: Other determinants

To better understand other social and cultural determinants of health, let's consider a case
study of the Ramu Nickel Mine in Papua New Guinea, owned by the Chinese company,
Metallurgical Corporation of China (MCC). In August 2019, 200,000 litres of toxic slurry from
the nickel mine spilt into the sea. You can read more information in this report, 'Chinese-
owned nickel plant spills waste into Papua New Guinea bay', by Reuters, a reputable global
news organisation, written at the time the incident happened: https://www.reuters.com/article/
us-papua-mining-spill-idUSKCN1VI0VW. It is several years now since this incident. Beyond
the immediate health and planetary concerns and calls for better management of mining waste
to avoid further spills, there are concerns about the long-term health impacts of heavy metals,
such as immune and nervous system disorders and cancer. However, in incidents like these,
there are other determinants of health, for example, the social and cultural determinants of
health such as the impact on traditional lifestyles. Do you think the mining companies like
MCC should be mandated to submit for approval, a health impact assessment of other
determinants of health such as social and cultural determinants of health?

Public health has always acknowledged war is political and bad for human and planetary health. Beyond ideology, it is fundamentally about resources: human, built, and environmental. The Russian-Ukrainian conflict, which started in February 2022 has recently re-ignited the debate about nuclear energy. In particular, the Zaporizhzhia Nuclear Power Plant, currently occupied by Russia, is at risk of a nuclear disaster. For many countries, including Australia and the US, nuclear power is a contested option in a diverse and futuristic national energy portfolio. There are issues related to the management of accidents, security, waste, and pollution and concerns for the natural environment. In the US, the Nuclear Regulatory Commission (NRC) is responsible for licensing nuclear power plants and has the power to consider SDG 12. As part of this process, the power plant must submit an environmental assessment as the baseline for NRC to draft an Environmental Impact Statement. Burger, Clarke, and Gochfeld (2011) outline types of ecological, fate and transport, and human health information required to evaluate the risk of safe sites for nuclear facilities. Ecological information includes biodiversity, ecosystems, habitats, landscapes and common, abundant, unique, endangered and rare species. Information for fate and transport includes potential sources of release for radionuclides and chemicals, the nature of these releases (e.g., subsurface liquids) and the features and properties of environmental media (such as groundwater chemistry, hydraulic gradient, wind speed). Human health information includes at-risk populations (e.g., demographics, distance), potential pathways (such as sources of drinking water) and exposure opportunities (lifestyle activities). The authors suggest stakeholders agree on a suite of site-specific indicators.

Indigenous perspective

Napandee, a remote locality in South Australia, located between Kimba and Hawker, is designated to be Australia's first nuclear waste site. The Barngarla Determination Aboriginal Corporation and the Barngarla people informed the cultural heritage management plan which ensures there is no disturbance of cultural heritage. However, Kimba locals cast a non-binding vote in favour of the nuclear waste site. The Barngarla native title group brought a case against the federal government to stop the proposed Nappanee nuclear waste site and lost. This report raises issues about the cultural determinants of health. Local community members from all ages and cultural backgrounds contributed to protest artworks. Local women spoke with Madeleine King, the Federal Resources Minister, who has the power to veto the site. They described how the waste dump would contravene the cultural heritage management plan by interfering with a sacred site for women. Here is a report: 'Barngarla women warn Kimba nuclear waste plan will 'destroy' sacred site, dreaming stories' (ABC North and West SA, 2023): https://www.abc.net.au/news/2023-03-05/barngarla-women-protest-against-nuclear-waste-at-kimba/102053982
What is the cultural impact of going ahead with the site on Aboriginal women in Kimba? What would be a strength-based approach to inform this discussion and decision?

Fashion

The fashion industry contributes to waste in terms of consumption and production, and consumers and citizens are challenging the industry. Have you heard of ethical fashion? There are lots of ethical dimensions to fashion, including a living wage for those who make our clothes. Note: labour costs are a small percentage of overall production cost. There is clear and strong market pressure on fashion brands to rethink supply chains. There is a significant push from citizens for fashion brands to actively address ethical issues in the long and complex supply chain, such as human rights and carbon offsets, with clear links to human health outcomes. This starts with a conscious examination of humanitarian and planetary principles, a financial commitment and significant injection of time. Oxfam, a not-for-profit organisation in the UK, started a *name and shame* approach called *Naughty or nice* to proactively progress change. The programme identifies fashion brands which have made improvements to address ethical production, and publicly shame those who could do better. Brands are required to verify commitments made to addressing supply chain exploitation. Brands such as JeansWest and Zara were shamed because they did not take action, or it could not be verified, or make commitments to a living wage. Brands such as Lorna Jane have made a commitment to at least analyse their wage gap.

'Fast fashion' (low-cost fashion in the latest styles) lends itself to ethical issues such as the cost of living because of small margins and profits. Hypothetically, the cost to a fashion brand of implementing a living wage would add 1% to the cost of a fashion item. That's 10c for a $10.00 t-shirt. However, the impact it could have on human's health could be significant. Fast fashion has sped up so quickly in the last two decades, it is now referred to as ultra-fast fashion. The industry has adapted by decreasing lead time and implementing smaller production cycles. It has never been so easy to buy cheap clothing, and this has changed the value of and the way we think about fashion. In Australia, approximately 200,000 tons of clothing and textiles end up in landfill every year, and potentially contributing to poorer human and planetary health outcomes. Papasolomou, Melanthiou and Tsamouridis (2023) investigated customers' (n = 97) levels of knowledge, attitudes, and behaviour toward fast fashion sustainability. Most consumers stated they know about fast fashion sustainability and women are more knowledgeable than men. Most consumers do not have detailed and correct knowledge about the supply chain. Men are willing to pay a higher price for fast fashion brands. The authors concluded that a shift to more sustainable fashion consumption is premised on strong feelings elicited by clear information about the environmental and social impact of products. This may force the fashion industry to respond to consumer demands.

Thinking about fashion, ask yourself these questions: How long have you owned the clothes you are wearing today? How many sets of clothes do you own? How much did they cost? Are they designer brands, such as Gucci or cheap fakes? Are they a staple item in your wardrobe? Do you buy good quality clothes to last or poor quality, on-trend clothes from low-cost chains? If you answered *poor quality, on-trend clothes from low-cost chains* to the last question, you are contributing to the fast fashion industry. Globally, the fast fashion industry produces 100 billion garments each year and one-third to three-quarters (estimates vary) of these garments end up in landfill, with consequences for human and planetary health, less than one year after purchase. Now, ask yourself this question: do you buy good quality clothes, clothes which will last a long time, or clothes from second-hand and op-shops? This is the sustainable 'slow fashion' industry.

Spotlight: Advocacy action

As a consumer, how could you advocate for more sustainable and ethical fashion and ultimately improve health and planetary outcomes? Let's think about fast and slow fashion and use a cocktail dress or a dinner suit as an example. The first question you should yourself is: *Do I need to buy a new cocktail dress or dinner suit, or do I need to buy it at all?* If so, you should think about what material it is made from – organic versus non-organic, natural versus synthetic, primary versus recycled, a monoculture-sourced cloth or a blend? And how it was made (e.g., were the machinists paid a living wage)? You should also consider if it can be reused, repaired or recycled. Or you could ask, *Could I rent it, borrow it, or find a second-hand cocktail dress or dinner suit?* Could you take part in a clothes swap or find something in the community free-box?

Do you think recycled fashion is good for the planet? Consumers are frequenting op-shops or accessing the high street free box. Some fashion brands are actively implementing strategies to be more environmentally friendly. Examples include making new garments from off cuts or producing active wear made from plastic bottles. According to the 2019 Parliamentary Enquiry into Waste Management and Recycling, the average Australian purchases 27kg of clothing and disposes of 23kg to landfill each year. Compared to 15 years ago, Australian purchase 60% more clothing items and throw them out twice as quickly. Think about the politics of production – should governments do something and what are the implications for SDG 12 targets. But does recycled equal sustainable? Think about this: It is easier to recycle plastic bottles to plastic bottles than to a polyester fibre because recycling a plastic bottle to a polyester fibre shortens its life cycle and uses more energy. While the industry claims sustainability, this is in direct conflict with profitability. Twenty years ago, the fashion industry produced 50 billion garments and pairs of shoes. Today, it's 120 billion. This increased production puts pressure on land, water and chemical use and impacts carbon emissions, affecting human and planetary health outcomes. However, the necessary system changes to produce fashion within planetary boundaries will require global citizenship and activism and policy.

Let's think

Do you think there is such a thing as fashion politics or fashion diplomacy? Let's deconstruct this fun idea by using an example. At the recent Pacific Island forum, US President Joe Biden gifted the Fijian Prime Minister, Frank Bainimarama a pair of Aviator sunglasses. President Biden has worn this brand of sunglasses since he was 18 years old and now they are a trademark of his personal style. Referred to as Biden-Aviators, they are said to symbolise strength, militarism and masculinity. After the meeting, photos of Biden and Bainimarama wearing Biden-Aviators were tweeted and symbolised celebrating with a friend, as 'on the same page' and sharing the same views. This phenomenon is known as fashion diplomacy. In fact, the Pacific Islands engaged in fashion diplomacy long before it had a name. Pacific Island leaders have a long tradition of wearing 'cultural' shirts from the host country at the Asia-Pacific Economic Cooperation (APEC) meeting along with other international guests. Find a photo of a regional meeting where an Australian Prime Minister is wearing a cultural shirt. Who is in the photo? Who is, and isn't, wearing a cultural shirt? Do you think fashion politics plays a role in shaping and strengthening regional unity and politics, for example, in the aftermath of Cyclone Yasa in 2020? Or is it just symbolic?

Water: The health impacts of the politics of water and water policy

A human right

The human body requires water for survival; without any water intake, death can occur within three days. Bodily functions enabled by water intake include metabolism, cell function, and regulation of body temperature and circulation (Armstrong & Johnson, 2018). A human becomes dehydrated when they lose 3% of their bodily fluids; an 8% loss can cause death (Shaheen et al. 2018). Freshwater use is so important to human existence that it is identified as one of nine 'planetary boundaries' that provide a 'safe operating space for humanity based on the intrinsic biophysical processes that regulate the stability of the Earth System' (Steffen et al., 2015, p. 1). Unlike other boundaries 'beyond the zone of uncertainty', including nitrogen and phosphorous flows and genetic diversity, freshwater is determined currently to be 'safe' and within planetary boundaries but evaluations identify the need for the balance of above- and below-ground water extraction to stay within sustainable limits for human and eco-system needs (Steffen et al., 2015). As water is central to human existence, it is therefore a basic human right. The opening quote to this chapter is taken from the UN's General Assembly resolution to recognise 'the right to safe and clean drinking water and sanitation as a human right that is essential for the full enjoyment of life and all human rights' (UN, 2010). This ambition has been incorporated into SDG 6 which details the importance of safe and affordable drinking water, prevention of water pollution, reparation and protec-tion of freshwater supplies, and 'transboundary cooperation' of water sources. SDG 6 also details effective wastewater management and treatment to achieve hygienic outcomes and expand opportunities for efficient reuse and recycling of this critical resource (UN, 2015b). These SDG 6 targets will be considered throughout this chapter in relation to protecting and upholding human health despite the political and other pressures on water and was-tewater resources.

Global context

Transboundary challenges around water are clearly described in the multi-nation reliance on the River Nile that passes through Ethiopia, Sudan and Egypt. The core of this conflict is described in a 2019 publication from the International Crisis Group, an international thinktank that seeks to 'prevent wars and shape policies that will build a more peaceful world'. The ICC wrote:

> Ethiopia is moving ahead with construction of Africa's largest dam, despite Egypt's worry that it will reduce the downstream flow of the Nile, the source of around 90 per cent of its freshwater supply. It is crucial that the parties resolve their dispute before the dam begins operating. **Why does it matter?** The Nile basin countries could be drawn into conflict because the stakes are so high: Ethiopia sees the hydroelectric dam as a defining national development project; Sudan covets the cheap electricity and expanded agricultural production that it promises; and Egypt perceives the pos-sible loss of water as an existential threat. **What should be done?** The three countries should adopt a two-step approach first, they should build confidence by agreeing upon terms for filling the dam's reservoir that do not harm downstream countries. Next, they should negotiate a new, transboundary framework for resource sharing to avert future conflicts.
>
> (ICC, 2019, p. i)

Despite Australia being a wealthy country, not all residents can turn on the kitchen tap and get safe and palatable drinking water. Consider remote Indigenous communities. Drinking water is the responsibility of specific utilities yet, in research describing the main-tenance of water and other essential services, householders reported they had minimal agency to effect change and long waiting periods and substandard services (Hall, 2019). This status of services for a geographically, racially and economically disadvantaged minority population does not align with Australia's commitment to the UN Declaration on the Rights of Indigenous Peoples (2007).

Indigenous perspective

A 2020 short film created by two Aboriginal women, Professor Sandra Creamer AO (Waanyi Kalkadoon) and Wendy Anders (Arrernte) sought to document Aboriginal women's experiences of remote living, and how essential services can affect the health of their families. One resident spoke to camera about drinking water, stating:

> We don't have a proper water supply out here … We access drinking water from a rainwater tank. In a drought, we have to buy 10 litre water cartons from town. We use bore water for washing clothes and for showers. It's salty water straight from the ground. The Government doesn't listen to us …
>
> (resident, Williams Well homeland, Northern Territory, in NATSIWA &UQ, 2020)

This experience of poor water access, security and acceptability is experienced in many parts of remote Australia. There are over 1,100 remote settlements in Australia where the population is majority Aboriginal and/or Torres Strait Islander Peoples. The tap water in over 500 of these remote settlements is not regularly tested and often not safe to drink (WSAA, 2022).

Acceptability of drinking water is critical to water consumption. While water may be evaluated as passing drinking water standards and thus 'potable' (safe to drink), it may not be 'palatable' (acceptable to drink) due to the colour, odour, taste or feeling on the skin and hair, and residue on appliances. The rejection of drinking water can have unintended health consequences, including dehydration or increased sugar intake through preferring consumption of sugar-sweetened beverages ('soft drinks' or 'sodas') contributing to weight gain, increased blood sugar levels and dental decay (Hall et al, 2021).

Contamination

Water and wastewater management are politically recognised as crucial for health protection. However, this resource is at risk of contamination and mismanagement that in turn creates a risk to human health. There are three main causes of water contamination: microbial, chemical and industrial. Microbial contamination of drinking water can be caused by bacteria, viruses and protozoa. The most common and widespread source of pathogenic contaminants is from human or animal faecal waste in the water source (NHMRC, 2018). The health impacts of these enteric ('from the gut') pathogens can range from mild (treatable diarrhoea) to severe (dysentery, hepatitis, cholera or typhoid fever) (NHMRC, 2018). To place this contamination in perspective of human health impact, diarrhoea (a common outcome from drinking microbially contaminated water) causes 3% of total disability-adjusted life years (DALYs) of 369 diseases and injuries (IHME, 2022).

Let's do

The acronym 'NTDs' refers to 'Neglected Tropical Diseases'. The World Health Organisation lists 20 NTDs caused by a variety of pathogens, including viruses, bacteria, parasites, fungi and toxins that affect the morbidity and mortality of over 1 billion people. Here is the link: https://www.who.int/news-room/questions-and-answers/item/neglected-tropical-diseases. In small groups, locate the WHO's list of 20 NTDs and, from the longer list, identify which of these diseases are waterborne ('the cause'). Map locations around the world where these preventable waterborne diseases occur. Which diseases can be reduced or eliminated through the availability of safe drinking water and adequate sewage treatment ('the prevention')? Discuss the terminology of 'neglected' diseases: What does this imply? Why are these diseases neglected when they affect one-eighth of the world's population? Discuss difficult issues of power, political attention, and the 'invisibility' created by poverty – all of which (and more) can affect where funding and public health efforts are directed to eliminate or prevent these diseases.

Drinking water sourced from under the ground ('aquifers', 'groundwater', 'artesian water') can be high in naturally occurring chemicals such as uranium, magnesium, nitrates and arsenic, due to rock geology and therefore unsafe for human consumption (Hall et al., 2021). Industrial contamination also impacts water sources, including from mining, military and agricultural sources. These contaminants include agricultural pesticides, excess (or mobilisation of) salt and high nutrient effluent (wastewater) (NHMRC, 2018). The treatment of these forms of pollution is specific to the contaminant but covered under the broad ambition in SDG 6, target 6.3 for 'reducing pollution, eliminating dumping and minimising release of hazardous chemicals and materials' (UN, 2015b). The financial and technical capability to treat these water source risks is spelt out in the UN's human right to water and sanitation.

Water security

A key term when considering the protection of water sources for human use, including consumption, is 'water security'. This can be defined as the ability of a nation/population to sustainably maintain sufficient quality and quantity of water for the needs of health and wellbeing, livelihoods and socio-economic development. Challenges to water security can be environmental (such as the impacts of droughts on water storage recharge), industrial (such as the tension between extractive and manufacturing needs, environmental needs and local population needs), and civil (including conflicts where water sources, such as rivers, flow across national or other jurisdictional borders). Ensuring safe and secure supplies of drinking water to enable populations to maintain their health and hygiene is a challenge for growing urban populations under climate change. In parallel, the treatment of sewage is very water-intensive, from the flushing of toilets to the processing of this waste and ultimate disposal or reuse. In response, some jurisdictions have moved to 'potable reuse': the recycling of water from treated sewage and stormwater to augment drinking water supplies (NHMRC, 2008).

In Southeast Queensland, Australia, dam levels of water supplies were dropping and severe water restrictions were in place during the 11-year-long 'millennium drought'. With no certain end to the drought, infrastructure for indirect potable reuse was installed, known as the Western Corridor Project. The treated wastewater was termed 'indirect' as it was mixed with other water sources so was only one component of the water supply. This project was intended to be established through a plebiscite, but the state government proceeded without this public vote. This decision was based in part on previous surveys during the drought that found high levels (over 70%) of societal support for 'purified recycled water' (Radcliffe, 2010). The recycled component was to be added to the water supply when the main storage dam dropped below 40% levels. The Western Corridor Project policy decision was made rapidly then rainfall occurred shortly afterwards in parallel with increasingly negative media coverage of the safety of the treatment technology and the general concept of recycled wastewater (Radcliffe, 20108). A prominent campaign against potable reuse, 'Citizens against Drinking Sewage', was led by a group based in a rural Queensland community and attracted significant media attention (Dolnicar et al., 2010). This affected societal perceptions and support in subsequent surveys that found Australians preferred desalinated water over recycled drinking water.

Let's do

Singapore has addressed its challenge of minimal drinking water sources through recycling wastewater. This water extraction process called 'indirect potable reuse' and has been a core component of Singapore's drinking water since 2003. To learn more, access public-facing documents about the benefits of 'NEWater' in Singapore (https://www.pub.gov.sg/watersupply/fournationaltaps/newater) and explore how the communication of this water security approach is delivered to the public. What are the key positive messages communicated about NEWater? How is the involvement of sewage in the production of drinking water communicated? What health risks are identified, and how are the risk management responses communicated? What are the political aspects behind the support and implementation of NEWater?

The Indo-Pacific region has a range of current and projected challenges to water security, with potential for regional conflict. This includes freshwater supplies negatively affected by climate change, a 'lack of direction' in transboundary cooperation of shared water catchments (watersheds), and insufficient funding of water security support (Ojha & Schofield, 2022). The political nature of civil conflict has direct impacts on human health in terms of providing stable, safe and sufficient water to meet the needs for humans and livelihoods. The physical environment of water requires upstream protection (literally!). Ensuring safe drinking water for human health starts far upstream from the kitchen tap.

Spotlight: Advocacy action

A world-first political process to protect the upstream features of drinking water can be seen by New Zealand's 2017 approach to assign equivalent human rights to a river (O'Donnell & Talbot-Jones, 2018). This approach recognised that innovative approaches were required to manage the health and ecological aspects of freshwater resources. Granting 'legal personhood' to a natural feature enables the legal rights, duties and responsibilities to be upheld by law (O'Donnell & Talbot-Jones, 2018). After many years of seeking to protect the Whanganui River from mismanagement and resource extraction, the Māori Traditional Owners, Whanganui Iwi (tribe), settled negotiations with the New Zealand Government (the Crown) with the establishment of the Te Awa Tupua (Whanganui River Claims Settlement) Act 2017. This Act provides legal personhood to the river and a guardian was appointed to the river to ensure the river's health and well-being. This and similar approaches in India and Australia have enabled freshwater conflicts regarding economic, cultural, environmental and management aspects to be addressed.

Environmental flow

One way in which water-based ecosystems are protected for human health and other needs is through ensuring sufficient water is in the natural system to maintain a balanced ecology. For rivers, this is known as 'environmental flows' and commonly defined as 'the quantity, timing, and quality of water flows required to sustain freshwater and estuarine ecosystems and the human livelihoods and well-being that depend on these ecosystems' (Brisbane Declaration, 2007). Environmental flows have proven politically controversial, as this brings a sharp focus onto society's diverse priorities for water. One example of environmental flow negotiations is around ecological management of the Snowy River in the states of New South Wales and Victoria in Australia. The Snowy Mountains Hydro-Electricity Scheme was constructed between 1949 and 1974 for electricity generation and some irrigation. This resulted in the diversion of up to 99% of the Snowy River's natural (environmental) flow. The significantly reduced river flow changed the water temperature to much lower due to deeper locations behind the dam wall, and much higher in shallow areas below the dam; combined with the unnatural timing of dam releases, this affected the breeding cycles of native fish and insects as well as the type and location of native vegetation and the presence weed and algal species (NSW Government, 2010).

Spotlight: Policy process

In response to public debate, the Snowy Water Inquiry was commissioned in 1998. It was charged to investigate environmental issues caused by the water diversion and propose

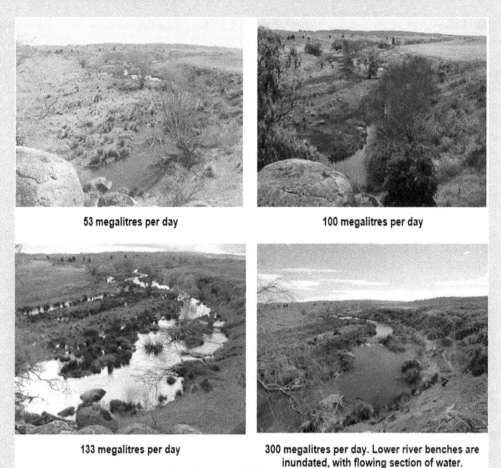

53 megalitres per day

100 megalitres per day

133 megalitres per day

300 megalitres per day. Lower river benches are inundated, with flowing section of water.

Figure 7.1 A bend in the Snowy River over time
Source: NSW Government (2010).

options that addressed environmental, economic and agricultural impacts (NSW Government, 2010). Environmental flow regimes have since been legislated. This example shows how political determinants – and the resulting policy changes – can affect an essential resource for human health in both negative and positive ways, as seen in Figure 7.1. There is visible ecological recovery of the Snowy River (downstream of Blackburn Creek and Dalgety, NSW) from increased environmental flows and removal of weed tress.

Let's finish

This chapter has highlighted some of the salient issues associated with waste and water from a political perspective and within the context of planetary health. As global populations modernise and urbanise, more and more complex waste is generated, accelerating the already overwhelming challenge of waste management. The first half of this chapter discussed single-use plastic, batteries, nuclear power and fashion and the impact on human health but the problem of waste and waste management is far from limited to these examples. Social movements, such as the circular economy, are gaining some momentum but are unlikely to impact consumption and consumer behaviour in the short term. The wide adoption of the circular economy will be slow and potentially tedious, given any tangible and enduring change will need to navigate vested interests and highly political local and global environments. However, there are significant imperatives for individuals, communities, organisations and governments at all levels to invest in innovative technological and biodiverse solutions or risk human and planetary health.

The second half of this chapter emphasises how water is required for human survival and is a basic human right explicated in the UN Sustainable Development Goal 6. Transboundary challenges are discussed before highlighting that not all people who live in Australia have access to 'potable' (safe) drinking water. Acceptability, that is, 'palatability' of drinking water is explored. The three main causes of water contamination (microbial, chemical and industrial) are examined. Water security is defined and considered by looking at the example of Southeast Queensland, Australia, during the 11-year-long 'millennium drought'. This section closes with a conversation about environmental flows in the natural water-based ecosystem, using the example of the Snowy Water Inquiry that investigated environmental impacts caused by the water diversion for hydroelectricity. This example highlights how policy changes can influence the political determinants of human and planetary health in both negative and positive ways.

Summary

In this chapter, you have gained a detailed understanding of a selection of contemporary and politicised issues associated with waste and water. This in-depth look provides you with insight into the complex nature of these issues and brings to the fore future challenges to protect planetary and human health.

After reading the chapter, you should now be able to:

• Understand household waste production and approaches to recycling, reusing and revaluing household waste. This chapter considered household consumption, before discussing recycling, reusing and revaluing with examples of single-use plastic, batteries and human waste. It problematised infrastructure and waste management within politics and future policy settings.

- Critique approaches to managing commercial waste including landfill and the circular economy from a planetary perspective. This chapter highlighted the specific commercial issues such as landfill and used nickel mining and nuclear energy as example of potential toxic waste. The circular economy was introduced. Commercial waste was situated within a political context, and the impact on the cultural determinants of health was considered.
- Critically analyse the ethics and sustainability of the fast fashion and slow fashion industry. The chapter flagged the rapidly rising problem of fast fashion, complex supply chains, and considered potential break points. It introduced an old idea of slow fashion and challenged you to think about ethical and sustainable fashion and your fashion behaviour.
- Recognise the challenges of delivering safe and acceptable drinking water and wastewater treatment now and in a climate-affected future. This chapter highlighted water is a human right and essential for human existence.
- Evaluate aspects of essential service water and wastewater delivery affected by political decisions. This chapter considered unsafe water is a preventable cause of disease and the 'invisibility' of poverty from political priorities and adequate funding.
- Synthesise features of water and wastewater management beyond technological solutions to include social, financial and cultural aspects. This chapter explored the difficulty of transboundary water management, the imperatives for the protection of freshwater sources within economic, social and political contexts and detailed existing sustainable initiatives for water security.

Tutorial exercises

1   Most of us consume plastic, but here's the big question – can Australian do better at recycling plastic? In small groups, think about how well your household recycles? Does your household recycle hard plastic, soft plastic, white glass, tin, aluminium or batteries? Does your household upcycle, repurpose or reuse? Could your household do better, and if so, what systems or structures would make it easier to recycle? Sketch out a one-page policy brief to submit to your local MP presenting your strategies to make household recycling easier.

2   Fashion, or at least clothing, is part of our daily lives. Let's think about this from a waste perspective. Organise your tutorial group into two smaller and roughly equal teams. Each team will debate one side of the topic 'the pros and cons of fast fashion verse the pros and cons of slow fashion'. Teams should discuss and construct their argument and any rebuttal points.

3   You are a public health expert on drinking water and wastewater treatment returning to Australia after several years working overseas. You are seeking to identify the latest priority issues in Australia as quickly as possible. Firstly, access the most recent national water and wastewater industry conference programme, OzWater (from the Australian Water Association). Now, find three presentations and posters on the program in these categories: technical, social/behavioural, political, financial, other. For each, summarise the pertinent issue in one sentence.

4   You have been engaged by the Pacific Community (SPC; https://www.spc.int/about-us) to support planning for drinking water on rural parts of Pacific islands. You meet with the SPC Water and Sanitation Programme team at their headquarters in New Caledonia. In preparation, access the WHO's small community water guidance tool for planning. Identify if this tool is relevant for Pacific Island Countries and Territories to produce potable AND palatable water. Also identify what baseline data you will need to collect before you commence planning the drinking water system.

Acknowledgements

Thank you to Ferne Edwards for her help in writing this chapter.

Further reading

Australian Government. Department of Climate Change, Energy, the Environment and Water. (2023). Environment protection. Available at: https://www.dcceew.gov.au/environment/protection

Chen, L., He, L., Yan, X. & Liu, C. (2022). Green message framing in enhancing sustainable consumption behavior of fashion based on the cross-theoretical model. *Journal of Environmental and Public Health*, 4038992. https://doi.org/10.1155/2022/4038992

Ruzhylo, S., Zakalyak, N., Ivanikiv, N., Popovych, D., Ƶukow, X. & Popovych, I. (2022) Features of EEG & HRV in 1997 in humans exposed to the factors of the accident at the Chornobylian nuclear power plant in 1986. *Journal of Education, Health and Sport*, 12(10), 214–224. http://dx.doi.org/10.12775/JEHS.2022.12.10.025

United Nations. (2015a). Sustainable Development Goals. Goal 12: Ensure sustainable consumption and production patterns. Available at: https://www.un.org/sustainabledevelopment/sustainable-consumption-production/

United Nations. (2015b). Sustainable Development Goals. Goal 6: Ensure access to water and sanitation for all. Available at: https://www.un.org/sustainabledevelopment/water-and-sanitation/

References

Armstrong, L. E., & Johnson, E. C. (2018). Water intake, water balance, and the elusive daily water requirement. *Nutrients*, 10(12), 1928. https://doi.org//10.3390/nu10121928

Brisbane Declaration. (2007). Environmental flows are essential for freshwater ecosystem health and human well-being. Paper presented at 10th International River Symposium and International Environmental Flows Conference, Brisbane, Australia. Available at: https://www.conservationgateway.org/ConservationPractices/Freshwater/EnvironmentalFlows/MethodsandTools/ELOHA/Pages/Brisbane-Declaration.aspx (accessed 6 June 2023).

Burger, J., Clarke, J., & Gochfeld, M. (2011). Information needs for siting new, and evaluating current, nuclear facilities: Ecology, fate and transport, and human health. *Environmental Monitoring and Assessment*, 172, 121–134. https://doi.10.1007/s10661-010-1321-y

Carson, R. (1962). *Silent Spring*. Boston: Houghton Mifflin.

Consumer Product Safety Commission. (2018). Status Report on High Energy Density Batteries Project. Available at: www.cpsc.gov/s3fs-public/High_Energy_Density

Cook, E., Velis, C. A., & Cottom, J. W. (2022). Scaling up resource recovery of plastics in the emergent circular economy to prevent plastic pollution: Assessment of risks to health and safety in the Global South. *Waste Management and Research*, 40(12), 1680–1707. https://doi.org/10.1177/0734242X221105415

DFAT (Department of Foreign Affairs and Trade). (2018). Voluntary national review. Canberra: DFAT. Available at: http://dfat.gov.au/aid/topics/development-issues/2030-agenda/Pages/voluntary-national-review.aspx (accessed 6 June 2023).

Dolnicar, S., Hurlimann, A., & Grun, B. (2010). What affects public acceptance of recycled and desalinated water? *Water Research* 45(2), 933–943. https://doi.org/10.1016/j.watres.2010.09.030.

Earle, W., Spencer, R., McCausland, P., Futeran, J., Webster, P., & Leslie, G. (2023). Walgett's drinking water: Yuwaya Ngarra-li. Briefing paper. Sydney: University of New South Wales. Available at: https://www.igd.unsw.edu.au (accessed 30 May 2023).

Hall, N. (2019). Challenges of WASH in remote Australian Indigenous communities. *Journal of Water, Sanitation and Hygiene for Development*, 9(3), 429–437. https://doi.org/10.2166/washdev.2019.154.

Hall, N., Lee, A., Hoy, W., & Creamer, S. (2021). Five enablers to deliver safe water and effective sewage treatment to remote Indigenous communities in Australia. *Rural and Remote Health*, 21(2). https://doi.org/10.22605/RRH6565

ICC. (2019). Bridging the gap in the Nile Waters dispute. Africa Report No. 271. Brussels: International Crisis Group. Available at: https://icg-prod.s3.amazonaws.com/271-bridging-the-gap.pdf (accessed 2 June 2023).

IHME. (2022). GBD compare data visualization. Seattle, WA: Institute for Health Metrics and Evaluation, University of Washington. Available at: http://vizhub.healthdata.org/gbd-compare. (accessed 1 June 2023).

National Health and Medical Research Council. (2008). Australian Guidelines for Water Recycling: Augmentation of drinking water supplies. Canberra. NHMRC Environment Protection and Heritage Council Natural Resource Management Ministerial Council. Available at: https://www.waterquality.gov.au/guidelines/recycled-water#augmentation-of-drinking-water-supplies-phase-2 (accessed 6 June 2023).

National Health and Medical Research Council. (2018). Australian Drinking Water Guidelines 6 2011 (Version 3.5). Canberra: National Health and Medical Research Council. Available at: https://www.nhmrc.gov.au/sites/default/files/documents/reports/aust-drinking-water-guidelines.pdf. (accessed 2 June 2023).

NATSIWA & UQ. (2020). Central Desert women talk about their health, their housing and their Country. Brisbane: National Aboriginal and Torres Strait Islander Women's Alliance and the University of Queensland. Available at: https://youtu.be/-xnCMiO9oUM (accessed 7 June 2023).

NSW Government. (2010). Returning environmental flows to the Snowy River: An overview of water recovery, management and delivery of increased flows. Sydney: Department of Environment, Climate Change and Water. Available at: https://www.industry.nsw.gov.au/__data/assets/pdf_file/0006/143619/Returning-environmental-flows-to-the-Snowy-River.pdf (accessed 6 June 2023).O'Donnell, E. L., & Talbot-Jones, J. (2018). Creating legal rights for rivers: Lessons from Australia, New Zealand, and India. *Ecology and Society*, 23(1). https://www.jstor.org/stable/26799037.

Ojha, H., & Schofield, N. (2022). Climate change and water security in the Indo-Pacific region: Risks, responses, and a framework for action. Canberra: Australian Water Partnership.

Papasolomou, I., Melanthiou, Y., & Tsamouridis, A. (2023). The fast fashion vs environment debate: Consumers' level of awareness, feelings, and behaviour towards sustainability within the fast-fashion sector. *Journal of Marketing Communications*, 29(2), 191–209. https://doi:10.1080/13527266.2022.2154059

Radcliffe, J. (2010). Evolution of water recycling in Australian cities since 2003. *Water Science & Technology*, 2(4), 792–802. https://doi.org/10.2166/wst.2010.362.

Shaheen, N. A., Alqahtani, A. A., Assiri, H., Alkhodair, R., & Hussein, M. A. (2018). Public knowledge of dehydration and fluid intake practices: Variation by participants' characteristics. *BMC Public Health*, 18(1), 1346. https://doi.org/10.1186/s12889-018-6252-5.

Steffen, W., Richardson, K., Rockstrom, J., Cornell, S. E., Fetzer, I., Bennett, E. M., Biggs, R., Carpenter, S. R., de Vries, W., & Sörlin, S. (2015). Planetary boundaries: Guiding human development on a changing planet. *Science*, 347(6223). https://doi.org/10.1126/science.1259855

Syms, R., Taylor-Robinson, S. D., & Trovato, G. (2023). Circular medicine: Being mindful of resources and waste recycling in healthcare systems. *Risk Management and Healthcare Policy*, 16, 267–270. https://doi.org/10.2147/RMHP.S396667

Takefuji, Y. (2022). Greener technology of lithium batteries is needed for healthy humans and nature. *Ethics, Medicine and Public Health*, 20, 100744. https://doi.org/10.1016/j.jemep.2021.100744

UN (United Nations). (2007). *Declaration on the rights of Indigenous peoples*. New York: United Nations.

UN (United Nations). (2010). *The human right to water and sanitation (A/RES/64/292)*. New York: United Nations.

United Nations. (2015a). Sustainable Development Goals. Goal 12: Ensure sustainable consumption and production patterns. Available at: https://www.un.org/sustainabledevelopment/sustainable-consumption-production/

United Nations. (2015b). Sustainable Development Goals. Goal 6: Ensure access to water and sanitation for all. Available at: https://www.un.org/sustainabledevelopment/water-and-sanitation/

Vardoulakis, S. (2021). Reflections on climate change and the Australian health system. *Australian Health Review*, 45(1), 2–3. https://doi:10.1071/AHv45n1_ED2

WSAA. (2022). Closing the water for people and communities gap. Sydney: Water Services Association of Australia. Available at: https://www.wsaa.asn.au/publication/closing-water-people-and-communities-gap-review-management-drinking-water-supplies (accessed 7 June 2023).

8 Climate and Environment

Linda A. Selvey

It is unequivocal that human influence has warmed the atmosphere, ocean and land. Widespread and rapid changes in the atmosphere, ocean, cryosphere and biosphere have occurred.

(IPCC et al., 2021, p. 4)

Learning objectives

After studying this chapter, you should be able to:

1 Discuss planetary health – the impacts of the climate crisis and environmental destruction on health.
2 Analyse the links between politics and the climate crisis and environmental destruction.
3 Describe the influence of the fossil fuel and other extraction industries on climate and environmental policies in Australia and globally.
4 Debate the tension between some determinants of health and some climate and environmental protection policies.
5 Critically analyse the concept of intergenerational equity and what this means for current and future politics.

Snapshot

As of December 2022, the global average surface temperature over land and sea had increased by 1.15°C since pre-industrial times. Because of the capacity of the ocean to absorb heat, increases in temperatures over land are higher than over the sea and sea surface temperatures are rising globally, with major implications for marine ecosystems and our climate systems. This increase in global average temperatures has already resulted in an increase in the frequency, duration and intensity of heatwaves, bushfires, storms, droughts and floods, as well as increased intensity of hurricanes and cyclones and accelerating rises in sea levels. As global average temperatures increase, so will these impacts. The main drivers of climate change are increasing greenhouse gases (predominantly but not exclusively CO_2 and methane), resulting from the mining and combustion of fossil fuels (coal, oil and gas), agriculture, and land use change (deforestation and land clearing). In spite of the threat of climate change, global emissions continue to increase.

DOI: 10.4324/9781003315490-13

Let's begin!

Australia has a diverse and highly variable climate, and increasing global average temperatures are accentuating this variability, resulting in the increasing frequency and severity of extreme weather events. Having been shaped and cared for by Aboriginal and Torres Strait Islander peoples for tens of thousands of years, Australia's natural environment has been rapidly transformed since colonisation, resulting in loss of habitat and biodiversity as well as land and soil degradation. Generally speaking, successive Australian governments have failed to institute policies to protect our natural environment and to reduce emissions. It is clear that globally, as in Australia, current political and economic systems are failing humanity as well as other species. The climate crisis and environmental destruction are the ultimate political determinants of health, given the irreversibility of their impacts. The first section of this chapter will describe some of the health impacts of climate change. The second section will discuss some of the impacts of environmental destruction on health. The chapter also includes an appraisal of some of the political factors that have shaped Australia's failure to address these challenges, as well as the concept of intergenerational equity.

The health impacts of the politics of climate and climate policy

Human health

Global warming is already impacting on human health, with increasing morbidity and mortality from heatwaves, injury and death from extreme weather events, reductions in food security, changes in patterns of infectious diseases and negative impacts on mental health. As the Earth warms, and the climate events as described above increase further, the climate crisis will increasingly impact on human systems such as our economies and on the very systems that sustain life. The climate crisis is already a major factor in the sixth mass extinction event that is likely happening now, and its contribution to extinction is increasing with increasing global average surface temperatures (IPBES, 2019).

As global average surface temperatures increase, heat extremes also increase. As of 2020, when global average surface temperatures were 1°C higher than pre-industrial levels, heatwave events that would have occurred once every 10 years occurred 2.8 times more frequently, or around every 4 years and were 1.2°C hotter than they would have been without human-induced global warming. When global average surface temperatures reach 1.5°C above pre-industrial levels (likely to be some time before 2030), a once-in-10 years heat event will occur an estimated 4.1 times more often, or around once every 2.5 years, and they will be 1.9°C hotter (IPCC et al., 2021). Exposure to high temperatures can directly impact on health by causing heat exhaustion and heat stroke. Heat stroke, when the body's core temperature reaches dangerously high levels, is a health emergency and can be fatal. The body's attempts to cool itself also stresses people's hearts and lungs, and dehydration from sweating can cause kidney failure. Therefore, morbidity and mortality due to heat can present as exacerbations of cardiovascular, respiratory or kidney disease. Exposure to heat has also been known to cause deaths and illness due to exacerbation of diabetes as well as pre-term births (Ebi et al., 2021). Longden (2019) investigated the impact of heat on mortality across Australia using mortality data from 2006 to 2017. The author found that both extreme heat and higher-than-average temperatures that were not extreme were associated with increased mortality. The overall number of deaths on hot days that were not extreme was higher than on days of extreme heat, most likely because such days occurred more often.

Let's think!

In Figure 8.1 you will see that both socioeconomic and socio-political factors influence the level of exposure to climate impacts and also that climate impacts can influence socio-economic and socio-political factors. Think about how these climate impacts could influence the socioeconomic and political conditions in a high-income country such as Australia.

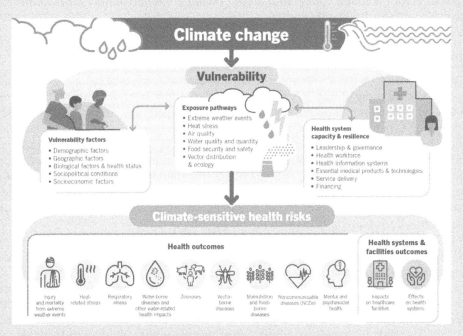

Figure 8.1 Risk pathways for the impacts of climate change on health
Source: World Health Organization (2021).

Indigenous perspective

In general, climate change disproportionally affects Aboriginal and Torres Strait Islander peoples in Australia compared to non-Indigenous Australians. Climate change exacerbates existing injustices such as inadequate housing and economic inequities. For example, people living in some remote communities are now being exposed to extreme heat while living in sub-standard housing with poor insulation. Low incomes and inadequate infrastructure mean that some people in these communities do not have access to fans or air-conditioning or even refrigeration during hot periods. Torres Strait Islander peoples living on low-lying islands in the Torres Strait are facing the threat of loss of their homelands as a consequence of sea-level rise. Aboriginal and Torres Strait Islander peoples have extensive local knowledge about their countries that can be harnessed for local solutions to the impacts of climate change. While many local solutions are being implemented, systemic racism means that Aboriginal and Torres Strait Islander peoples are not sufficiently being included in discussions about climate action.

An important local solution that has been taken up is the reinstatement of traditional burning practices across many parts of Northern Australia. Reinstating traditional burning is an important climate change mitigation strategy that has prevented significant amounts of CO_2 from being released into the atmosphere through wildfires. Traditional burning involves burning of small patches of the landscape during the cooler months. This promotes biodiversity and through fuel reduction also prevents large-scale hot fires. Being an important cultural practice across much of the Australian continent, supporting traditional burning also strengthens culture through caring for country. Funding through carbon credits also provides an income source for traditional owners.

The climate crisis

Scientific consensus on global warming and its causes was achieved at the Stockholm Convention in 1972 and the advice was formalised with the first Intergovernmental Panel on Climate Change (IPCC) report in 1990. With increasing temperatures and emissions, the level of knowledge of the urgency of the climate crisis continues to increase, but to date there is insufficient global action to address this crisis (Glavovic et al., 2021). Thus, it could be said that a failure to limit the extent of global warming due to human activity has been due to a failure of global politics to protect humanity and other life on Earth. This is in spite of many efforts by countries who stand to lose the most from the climate crisis, and by scientists and civil society to convince leaders of the world's richest nations to reduce their emissions. It begs the question: *why has humanity allowed this to happen?*

While individual action to reduce emissions is important, achieving the changes in the global economy to meaningfully address the climate crisis requires decisive policy action by governments throughout the world. It requires a commitment to emissions reduction targets and policy mechanisms to achieve the targets as well as financial contributions to support low- and middle-income countries to do the same. Some high-income countries particularly in Europe have led the way in emissions reduction and finance for global efforts to reduce emissions. Even so, while their emissions have fallen, they have not yet fallen to levels that would limit the probability of increases in global average temperatures beyond 1.5°C (IPCC et al., 2021). Australia's emissions continue to rise, and Australia is the world's largest exporter of gas and second largest exporter of thermal coal. While in most European countries, climate change is not considered to be an issue specific to either the Left or the Right of politics, in countries such as Australia, the USA and Canada, climate change is considered to be only an issue for the Left, with climate denial being more common on the Right. *Why do you think this might be so?* Indeed, Australia's climate policy has faced a rocky road in the past 30 years.

Global context

By its very nature, climate change is a global issue. The United Nations Framework Convention on Climate Change (UNFCCC) was set up 30 years ago as a mechanism to reach agreement between countries about how to address climate change, including seeking commitments by governments to reduce emissions and determining mechanisms for accountability. The fact that the impacts of climate change are not dictated by where the emissions came from has created tremendous inequities, as countries who have contributed the least to global warming also have the least capacity to adapt and respond due to their low incomes. Many of these countries have been vocal in UNFCCC meetings, including the annual Conference of the Parties (COPs), in calling for drastic measures to limit emissions as well as the provision of funding for mitigation, adaptation and for compensation for the unavoidable harms they have experienced and will experience as a result of the climate crisis.

The Green Climate Fund was set up under the auspices of the UNFCCC at COP16 in 2010 to support low- and middle-income countries in climate mitigation and adaptation. The fund relies on funding pledges by individual countries, which means it is vulnerable to changing politics in high income countries. A major strength of the Fund is that low- and middle-income countries own the projects for which they receive funding. In 2022, at COP27, an agreement was made to establish a Loss and Damage fund to compensate low- and middle- income countries for damages due to unavoidable climate risks (those that cannot be adapted to) arising from the activities of countries with the highest level of emissions. A Loss and Damage fund has been advocated for by many countries for a long time without success, and the agreement for the fund was long-awaited. Many details about the fund that could have ramifications for its success have yet to be agreed upon, however, but this is a major step forward.

Climate policy

Precipitated by the hosting of an international conference about climate change in Australia in the late 1980s, there was widespread Australian media coverage about climate change and its causes from then to the early 1990s. In 1990, Australia's then Labor Prime Minister announced an emissions reduction target of 20% below 1988 levels by 2005. However, a global recession and a change in Labor Prime Minister in 1991 reduced the impetus for action, which was cemented by a Liberal Prime Minister when he was elected in 1996. In 1997, under the Kyoto Protocol, the then Prime Minister successfully negotiated for an *increase* in Australia's emissions by 8% over 1990 levels, while refusing to ratify the Protocol. In 2012, a market-based carbon tax was introduced by the Labor Prime Minister who was in power with the support of the Greens. This led to a fall in emissions, but it was axed by a Liberal Prime Minister in 2014 (Crowley, 2021).

The next Liberal Prime Minister signed the UNFCCC Paris Agreement in 2017, with an inadequate emissions reduction target of 26–28% reduction of 2005 levels by 2030. Since 2014, Australia has not had an adequate mechanism to reduce emissions. Under another former Liberal Prime Minister, Australia failed to increase its climate ambition and was dubbed a 'climate denier' by international observers. During the eight-and-a-half-year period from September 2013 when Australia had a succession of Liberal Prime Ministers, there was also an unwritten policy within government of dismissing climate science. For example, the CSIRO, which formerly had a strong cadre of climate scientists, made significant cuts to jobs in climate science in 2016. In Australia, climate change was seen as a controversial and partisan issue.

In May 2022, in what has been dubbed by some as the 'climate election', Australian Labor party leader Anthony Albanese was elected as Prime Minister, alongside a record number of Greens and Independent candidates, all of whom were calling for increased climate action. Australia has increased its emissions reduction targets to a 43% reduction of 2005 levels by 2030, which is still inadequate according to the science. Many commentators believe that concern about climate change was an important factor in Labor's win. In spite of this, both major political parties in Australia, Labor and Liberal, support new coal and gas mines, including providing financial subsidies for some. This is counter to the expert evidence of the IPCC and other organisations that states that it is not possible to have a safe climate if new fossil fuel mines are opened. Because of this, many activists are involved in campaigns to stop new coal and gas mines in Australia, through legal challenges, shareholder action, attempts to delegitimise the fossil fuel industry and by targeting banks to stop them from financing new mines.

172   *Linda A. Selvey*

Let's do!

Go the Market Forces website: https://www.marketforces.org.au/ and look up your own bank and your Superannuation Fund if you have one. Do they fund the fossil fuel industry? Discuss this in your tutorial group. How many of you have some of your money in these institutions? Look at the range of campaigns in which Market Forces is involved. In your group, discuss the pros and cons of campaigns attempting to influence political decisions versus campaigns targeting financial institutions and businesses.

Fossil fuel industries

Australia's political and economic development has been dependent on coal since colonisation, and this has continued to the present day (Baer, 2016). In 2017/2018, Australia's fossil fuel exports (coal, oil and gas) were 24.5% of Australia's export income. Coal was Australia's second largest source of export income in that period (15%) second only to iron ore (15.2%). Being such a large part of the Australian economy results in power that is assumed rather than having to be regularly influenced (Stutzer et al., 2021).

The mining and fossil fuel industries also built on this power through directly lobbying governments and through influencing public opinion through advertisements. The latter has been reinforced in Australia through strong support of the fossil fuel industry by News Corp, which in 2019–2020 had almost 52% of the Australian newspaper market share. News Corp and major coal mining companies share investors and some major investment funds own large shares in both News Corp and major Australian coal mining companies (Stutzer et al., 2021). In one study, Stutzer et al. (2021) found that in the period leading to the approval of the Adani Carmichael Coal Mine in Queensland's Galilee Basin, the *Courier Mail*, Queensland's major newspaper, published numerous articles promoting the benefits of the mine and denigrating activists who were opposing it. This was in contrast to the news articles about the mine that were published by the Australian Broadcasting Commission, which had more emphasis on climate change, science and environmental impacts.

Spotlight: power dynamics: The power of lobbying

The fossil fuel industry also wields power through lobbying in Australia and globally. Lobbying is most effective when lobbyists have existing relationships with government ministers and experience in working in government. In Australia and elsewhere, certain individuals move between politics, lobbying firms and industry peak bodies. This results in increased access to meetings with government as well as an opportunity to build on and benefit from existing relationships. A report by the Grattan Institute (Wood et al., 2018) described an increasing number of registered lobbyists who were former government representatives (almost 40% of all lobbyists in 2018). One quarter of Australian government ministers or assistant ministers take on roles with special interests when they leave politics.

Lobbyists from the coal, oil and gas industry also attend the United Nations Framework Convention on Climate Change (UNFCCC) Conferences of the Parties (COP), even though these gatherings are focused on reducing emissions. For example, at the UNFCCC COP27, which was held in Egypt in November 2022, there were 636 lobbyists attending from the fossil fuel industry. These lobbyists attended as members of different country delegations. They outnumbered the delegates from each individual country attending, except for the United Arab Emirates.

Do you think that lobbyists from the fossil fuel industry should be allowed to participate in UNFCCC meetings? If not, how could that be stopped?

The power of the mining industry has also been used to discourage investment in renewable energy and boost fossil fuel subsidies while also influencing the public discourse about climate change. In the financial year 2021/2022, AUD 11.6 billion was spent by federal and jurisdictional governments on fossil fuel subsidies, with the majority of these subsidies (AUD 10.5 billion) being from the Federal government. While a large proportion of the Federal government subsidies (AUD 9.4 billion) were in the form of tax concessions (22% of which goes to the fossil fuel industry), the remainder was directly in support of fossil fuel mining or power stations. This compares to an estimated AUD 7.7 billion in subsidies to the renewable energy sector in the same time period (Armistead et al., 2022).

Professor Naomi Oreskes and Dr Eric Conway, both science historians, have documented the role of deliberate attempts to cast doubt on climate science as a way to stop policy action to reduce emissions. They drew comparisons with the role of doubt in slowing policy and regulation to reduce the harms of tobacco. The efforts to dispute climate science have largely been led by senior scientists who are specialists in fields other than climate science, and who work in institutes and think tanks that receive significant amounts of funding from the fossil fuel industry (Oreskes & Conway, 2010). The philosophy underpinning this denial seems to be about free markets, diminished role of government, and libertarianism. This denial has been promoted through direct relationships with politicians, and through the media. In addition, they have attacked individual scientists as well as institutions, such as the Intergovernmental Panel on Climate Change.

Spotlight: policy process: The ongoing role of ExxonMobil in slowing climate action

ExxonMobil is one of the world's largest public international oil and gas companies. As early as 1979, ExxonMobil published internal documents acknowledging the science of climate change and the significant effects that climate change will have on the environment. In spite of this acknowledgement, their public documents were less decisive and cast doubt on the severity of the changes, while also critiquing the science itself, and the scientists doing the work (Supran & Oreskes, 2017). ExxonMobil continues to promote misinformation about climate change and its solutions through advertising and advertorials while at the same time acknowledging climate science in their internal documents. Rather than outright denial, their rhetoric is more subtle. This rhetoric of doubt, in which climate change is acknowledged but minimised while at the same time espousing the virtues of the fossil fuel industry, is reflected in the current discourse about climate change in the USA and Australia. Supran and Oreskes (2017; 2021), who have analysed public and internal documents authored by ExxonMobil, describe their rhetoric as 'climate risk', 'consumer demand' and 'Fossil Fuel saviour'. Describing fossil fuels as increasing the risk of climate change, rather than as causing climate change downplays the role of fossil fuels in climate change. The rhetoric of 'consumer demand' blames individuals for their energy consumption rather than the fact that their energy supply is dominated by fossil fuels because of government inaction. The 'Fossil Fuel saviour' rhetoric refers to the role of fossil fuels in providing energy, jobs and economic growth, again assuming that fossil fuels are the only solution to energy needs. Through playing on the fundamental values of major political parties and the public, the above rhetoric has been particularly successful in halting progress on renewable energy and other measures to reduce emissions in countries such as the USA and Australia (Oreskes et al., 2018).

Learning activity: Let's think

What other industries have a large influence on political decision-making through the mechanisms described above? How many of these are advocating for policies that negatively affect health? What would need to happen to remove the level of power and influence that these industries have?

The health impacts of the politics of environment and environment policy

Biodiversity and ecosystems

The health effects of loss of biodiversity and ecosystem services are becoming increasingly apparent. Biodiversity supports humanity in many ways, including pollination of trees and crops, carbon capture and storage, providing novel sources of drugs, protecting water courses and providing spaces for curiosity, wonder, creativity and renewal (IPBES, 2019) (Figure 8.2). Ecosystem services is a term used to describe the many ways that our natural systems sustain human systems. Some examples of ecosystem services include pollination, carbon sequestration, protecting coastlines, reducing runoff during heavy rainfall, thus reducing the risk of flooding and contamination of water supplies, stabilisation of the water table, thus reducing soil salinity, and reducing air pollution. Air and water pollution are increasing, with consequent health impacts, as is land clearing, potentially releasing more CO_2 and methane into the atmosphere, and reducing the global capacity to absorb atmospheric CO_2. Pollinators, for example, insects, birds and flying foxes, are declining globally with consequences for food availability and forest regeneration. Studies have shown that the loss of pollinators has already resulted in a reduction of crop yields in countries across Asia, Africa and South and Central America. If this trend continues, there will be major consequences for nutrition and food security (Myers, 2020). Overfishing is resulting in the collapse of a number of fish stocks with consequent implications for ocean ecologies, human livelihoods and food. These changes are accelerating with increasing global population, consumption, economic growth and technological changes (IPBES, 2019). They are also increasing global inequities and threatening progress on the UN Sustainable Development Goals (IPBES, 2019). According to the Intergovernmental Science-Policy Platform on Biodiversity and Ecosystem Services (IPBES), 'transformative change across economic, social, political and technological factors' is required to address the accelerating loss of biodiversity and ecosystem services (IPBES, 2019, p. 14). These changes will require changes in policy and legislation at all levels of government, as well as in societal values and consumption patterns.

In Australia in April 2019, 100 plant and animal species were deemed to have been made extinct since European colonisation. There are now 1,918 species on the threatened or endangered list, and 19 Australian ecosystems are at risk of collapse. The greatest threat to biodiversity in Australia is habitat loss and degradation due to a range of ongoing activities including agriculture, logging, urbanisation, mining and transportation. Invasive species are also a major threat to biodiversity in Australia (Cresswell et al., 2021). Some impacts of the loss of ecosystem services in Australia include dryland salinity and soil erosion, with negative consequences for agriculture. *How important is biodiversity and ecosystem collapse to you? How much do you think Australia should curb industries and other human activity to protect biodiversity and ecosystems?*

Global perspective

It has been estimated that around 1 million species face extinction globally; many within the next decade. The rapidity and number of the extinctions suggests that we are likely at the start of the sixth mass extinction event on Earth, the previous one being due to an asteroid striking Earth around half a billion years ago. This, therefore, would be the only mass extinction event due to a single species, *Homo sapiens*. The largest cause of extinction globally is the clearing of land and forests, although climate change is increasingly playing a part. Land clearing and deforestation can occur as a result of deliberate policies, such as a deliberate policy of exploitation of the Amazon rainforests in Brazil that was introduced by the former Brazilian President Jair Bolsonaro. In other situations, land clearing occurs without policies to either protect or exploit the land, particularly on urban fringes and in rural areas, and is largely a result of population growth and/or land degradation. In order to solve these challenges and protect remaining biodiversity, global transformative change, as described by the IPBES, is necessary (IPBES, 2019).

Air pollution

It has been estimated that air pollution, including particulate matter, oxides of nitrogen, ozone, and sulphur dioxide, is responsible for over 4 million deaths per year globally. Most air pollution comes from combustion of fossil fuels and biomass, including during bushfires and burn offs, although dust is also an important source. In general, air quality in Australia is good by global standards. In spite of this, it has been estimated that air pollution in Australia is responsible for around 2,600 deaths per year. Air pollution can be irritating and can cause inflammation of the lungs and blood vessels and has been associated with increasing rates of asthma in Australia and elsewhere. It can also decrease exercise tolerance. In addition to asthma, exposure to air pollution can lead to increased cardiovascular events, lower respiratory tract infection, and chronic obstructive pulmonary disease. A recent systematic review of studies investigating the influence of air pollution on health has found that asthma and cardiovascular disease were important health impacts of air pollution in Australia (Walter et al., 2021).

Petrol- and diesel- powered cars and trucks are important sources of air pollution in Australia. Wood-burning heaters and stoves are also an important source, particularly in winter. The burning of fossil fuels for electricity and industry are also important sources, even though electricity and other industries that burn fossil fuels are usually located away from major urban centres. On the whole, Australian cities favour cars over public and active transport. Urban sprawl is Australia's response to population growth, and it results in land clearing for housing and road development. New housing developments are often built away from public transport corridors, resulting in increased car dependence for transportation. Apart from biodiversity loss from habitat destruction, increased road trauma and air pollution, long car commutes also decrease available time for family, physical activity, healthy eating and recreation. Planning decisions on new developments are made by state/territory and local governments in Australia and have proven to be difficult to influence or reverse. Part of this is cultural, with strong demand in Australia for large, detached houses.

Changes in drivers that indirectly affect biodiversity, such as population, technology, and lifestyle (upper right corner of Figure), can lead to changes in drivers directly affecting biodiversity, such as the catch of fish or the application of fertilizers (lower right corner). These result in changes to ecosystems and the services they provide (lower left corner), thereby affecting human well-being. These interactions can take place at more than one scale and can cross scales. For example, an international demand for timber may lead to a regional loss of forest cover, which increases flood magnitude along a local stretch of a river. Similarly, the interactions can take place across different time scales. Different strategies and interventions can be applied at many points in this framework to enhance human well-being and conserve ecosystems.

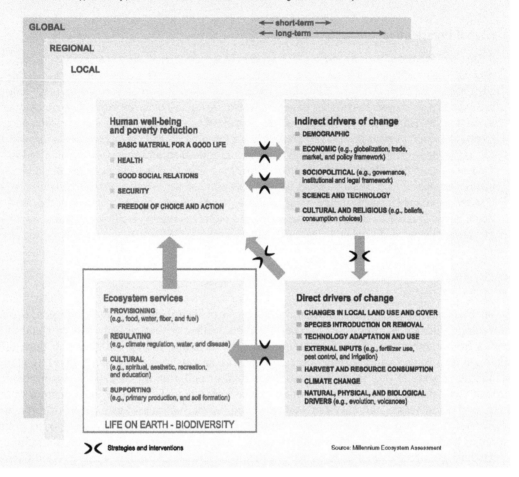

Figure 8.2 Conceptual framework of the interactions between biodiversity, ecosystem services, human wellbeing and drivers of change

Source: Millennium Ecosystem Assessment (2005), p. vii, Figure B. Copyright © 2005 World Resources Institute.

Mining

Apart from the existential threat of the climate crisis and air pollution, there are other direct health harms arising from mining. Coal mining can be harmful to coal miners. From 2007–2008 to 2011–2012, 36 mining workers died in Australia and there were 14.2 successful workers compensation claims for serious injury or illness per 1000 mining workers in Australia in 2011–2012 (Safe Work Australia, 2012). Coal mine dust lung disease is a serious condition that occurs following regular inhalation of fine particulate coal dust over a period of time. It can be debilitating and can lead to death. It was previously thought that this condition only occurred in underground coal mines, but recently it has been described in above ground coal mines as well. One study (Baade et al., 2021) estimated that, in 2020, 166 coal miners were diagnosed with coal mine dust lung disease in Queensland, with the majority of these having worked in surface mines since 2002. While coal mines are required to screen their workers for coal mine dust disease, until recently this was only required for workers in underground mines.

Mining not only has impacts on our climate, it also results in significant habitat destruction and ecosystem harm. One way that mining companies get around these environmental impacts is by 'offsetting', where they purchase land somewhere else that will be protected from destruction through this purchase. This approach is flawed but allowable under existing environmental protection legislation. Mining can also impact on water tables, potentially resulting in the loss or contamination of ground water, which is essential for ecosystems as well as farming and other uses. This can also lead to land subsidence. Coal mining itself is highly water-intensive, as water is used to wash the coal. Increasingly, water allocations to coal miners have angered local farmers who rely on water for their crops. The loss of ecological and cultural value of land is also an important impact that has created particular harm for Aboriginal and Torres Strait Islander peoples.

Spotlight: other determinants: The tension between potential health benefits of mining vs climate and environmental harms

Having a job, sufficient income, social connections, and access to safe housing and good food are intermediary determinants of health (World Health Organization, 2010). In Australia, jobs in the mining industry are generally well-paid, and some towns such as Moranbah in central Queensland have been built around coal mining. Others, such as many communities in Western Queensland, have had considerable injections of people and funds from gas mining, although in some cases this has decreased the affordability of housing for others not working in the industry. Coal mines previously supported local communities through funding schools and other infrastructure, although increasing use of fly-in fly-out models of staffing reduces that support (Stutzer et al., 2021). Around 46,400 people in Australia were employed in coal mining in 2022 (Australian Industry and Skills Committee, n.d.), and around 17,290 people were employed in oil and gas extraction in the 2020/2021 financial year (Statista, 2022). This is around 0.5% of all people employed in Australia in 2022 (Australian Bureau of Statistics, 2022). While, compared to other sectors that are dependent on a safe climate, such as tourism and agriculture, the number of jobs employed by the fossil fuel industry are few (and are often exaggerated), they are well-paid jobs in comparison to the other sectors, so those employed in the industry are not keen to give them up.

States and territories also receive valuable income from mining royalties. For example, in the financial year 2021/2022, the Queensland government received AUD 2.04 billion in royalties from coal and gas, by far the highest proportion of mining royalties in the state (Queensland Government, 2022). Also in the financial year 2020/2021, New South Wales received around AUD 1.5 billion in royalties from coal and gas, the vast majority of which came from coal (New South Wales Government, n.d.). Mining royalties contribute to the cost of providing healthcare, public health services, and education, all of which contribute to better health and wellbeing of the population. Mining royalties are, however, volatile, and are dependent on the price of these commodities in the international market.

While the fossil fuel industry might improve the health and wellbeing of some Australians, this is not distributed equitably across the population. Therefore, there is a tension between the current health and economic benefits of mining and the fossil fuel industry in Australia and the current and future harms of the industry due to its role in accelerating the climate crisis, increasing biodiversity loss and threatening water security.

Let's do

In your group, debate the following question: Does the Australian government's support of mining and the fossil fuel industry have overall positive or negative impacts on the health of Australians? For the debate, some students should support the proposition that mining has positive impacts and other students should support the proposition that mining has negative impacts on the health of Australians.

Indigenous perspective

Since the beginning of colonisation, Aboriginal and Torres Strait Islander peoples have resisted threats to their sovereignty and sought to protect their lands, countries and cultures. A healthy country is an important component of the health and wellbeing of Aboriginal and Torres Strait Islander peoples. The Aboriginal Land Rights (Northern Territory) Act 1976 and equivalent legislation in the Northern Territory convey ownership of the land where rights have been granted. Native Title legislation recognises the rights of Aboriginal and Torres Strait Islander peoples to their lands and sea but does not grant ownership. The Aboriginal Land Rights Act allows traditional owners to veto mining exploration and negotiate conditions, whereas the Native Title legislation allows for negotiation of conditions but with no veto power.

Intergenerational equity

In assessing the costs and benefits of a particular initiative, economists give a higher value to immediate compared to future costs and benefits. This is referred to as discounting. Economists also assess direct financial benefits and costs and rarely consider non-monetary costs and benefits. Discounting is effectively passing on to future generations the true costs of current human activity. This raises questions about whether current approaches to economics are ethical (Polasky & Dampha, 2021). Carbon pricing and other similar measures aim to take into account the true cost of fossil fuel combustion, thus levelling the playing field for renewable energy, which can have a high up-front cost.

The concept of intergenerational equity is based on a value of focusing on the rights of both present and future generations. Intergenerational equity means that the ability to meet the needs of future generations are not threatened by meeting the needs of current generations (Summers & Smith, 2014). Other concepts of equity are also important considerations in relation to climate and environmental policy. Currently there are considerable health and social inequities within Australia and other countries, and, on the whole, these are increasing. There is even greater inequity globally, and this is increasing as a result of the climate crisis and environmental destruction. One important consideration in relation to the climate crisis and mass extinction in relation to intergenerational equity is the irreversibility of many of many of the impacts of both crises in human timescales. CO_2 lasts in the atmosphere for thousands of years, and the earth will continue to warm even if no further greenhouse gases were emitted. Sea levels would continue to rise, and this rise, as well as glacial ice loss cannot be reversed for thousands of years. The rise in ocean temperatures and ocean dead zones also cannot be reversed for hundreds of years. Extinction is irreversible in any timeframe, and several other planetary boundaries, once traversed are also irreversible. At current emissions trajectories, the Earth will warm by at least 2.4°C by 2050 and 2.8 to 3.8°C by 2100, compared to pre-industrial times. Many scientists consider that this degree of warming would be incompatible with human civilisation (IPCC et al., 2021). Children born in 2022 will be 78 in 2100 if current estimates of life expectancy in Australia are realised, so, in effect, while intergenerational equity is often considered to refer to future generations, the climate crisis is also threatening current generations.

Equity is a fundamental value of public health, but there are few public health issues that require consideration of equity not just for the people who live now, but for future humanity and other species as well. The climate crisis, ecosystem destruction and biodiversity loss are three issues for which the concept of intergenerational equity is critical.

Let's do

As a result of human activity supported by government policies and global capitalism, the health and wellbeing of future generations is under threat. It can feel as though these policies and our economic system are too challenging to address. In your class, research some ideas that others have proposed to produce a significant change in the way that Australian and global economies operate and thus improve equity. Choose one such change. Discuss with each other how you could influence Australian and global politics to create this change.

Let's finish

Since colonisation, the politics of climate change and the environment in Australia is a reflection of the power of vested interests, particularly when aligned with mainstream white Australian values and the pursuit of economic growth. Australia's economy since colonisation was founded on resource extraction and agriculture, resulting in significant harm to the natural environment, soils and river systems. In recent years, technological changes have enabled more rapid and extensive land clearing and resource extraction, with consequent acceleration in environmental harms and carbon emissions.

This is reflected on a global scale, and, in spite of 30 years of the UNFCCC, global carbon emissions continue to rise. It seems as though humanity is unable or unwilling to change the systems that are driving the climate and biodiversity crises. This chapter describes some of the mechanisms by which vested interests have influenced politics to the detriment of current and future generations. Some of these mechanisms are public-facing, such as through advertising and discrediting experts, and some are directly targeted at decision-makers. Working within the systems that created these challenges is unlikely to result in the degree of transformation required to solve these global crises. Collective resistance, in its many forms may be the only answer.

Summary

This chapter describes some of the health impacts from climate and environmental changes. These changes are as a result of policy decisions, and lack of policy decisions, that have allowed and promoted these changes, in spite of their impacts.

Learning outcomes

After reading this chapter, you should now be able to:

- *Discuss planetary health – the impacts of the climate crisis and environmental destruction on health*: The chapter gives several examples of how the climate crisis and environmental destruction impact on health. The chapter also lists some of these changes that are irreversible in human timeframes. The chapter also shows how increasing global heating and biodiversity loss will increasingly impact on health and wellbeing.
- *Analyse the links between politics and the climate crisis and environmental destruction*: The chapter shows how both political action and political inaction in Australia and globally have resulted in continuing increases in greenhouse gas emissions and ongoing environmental destruction. Particularly in Australia, the political decision making in relation to greenhouse gas emissions and ongoing environmental destruction is linked to a history of reliance on resource extraction for its economy. The chapter also points out that major changes to human economic and social systems are required in order to minimise the impacts of the climate crisis and environmental destruction.
- *Describe the influence of the fossil fuel and other extraction industries on climate and environmental policies in Australia and globally*: The chapter illustrates some of the ways that fossil fuel and other extraction industries influences politics in Australia and globally. These industries use similar tactics to influence governments as other industries do, many of which also have a negative influence on health and wellbeing.
- *Debate the tension between some determinants of health and some climate and environmental protection policies*: Human health and wellbeing are influenced by economic factors such as employment and access to services that promote health and wellbeing. Some industries that harm our climate and environment also provide employment as well as government income that is spent on essential government services such as health. The chapter discusses this tension.
- *Critically analyse the concept of intergenerational equity and what this means for current and future politics*: Planning and acting to ensure equity for current and future generations, the concept of intergenerational equity, are what we should aspire to. However, our current economic system benefits the immediate needs of current generations at the expense of those coming after us. This chapter discusses the concept of intergenerational equity in the context of the climate crisis and biodiversity loss.

Tutorial exercises

1   This chapter has described some of the ways that human-induced global warming is impacting on weather patterns and sea level rise. Working in a small team identify some other potential health impacts of climate change and how they may manifest in high income country such as Australia as well as in low- and middle-income countries? Discuss these impacts in your group, particularly any differences between impacts in high income countries compared to low- and middle-income countries.

2   Imagine that you are two community leaders facing an angry community who have just been informed that a coal mine that they were expecting would result in local jobs and income for the community will not be going ahead because burning the coal from the mine will increase global emissions. One community leader supports the mine going ahead while the other one has campaigned to stop the mine because of its contribution to the climate

crisis. Divide your group into two teams. One team will take the side of the community leader supporting the coal mine and the other team will take the side of the community leader opposing the mine. Debate the issue from the perspectives of the community leaders. Each team should include the perspective of intergenerational equity in their discussion.

3   The IPBES has identified that global transformative changes are required to protect the remaining biodiversity and ecosystem services. Working in a small group, identify which major transformative changes would be needed in Australia to protect our remaining biodiversity and ecosystem services.

Further reading

Anderson, K. (2023). IPCC's conservative nature masks true scale of action needed to avert catastrophic climate change. *The Conversation*, 23 March. Available at: https://theconversation.com/ipccs-conserva tive-nature-masks-true-scale-of-action-needed-to-avert-catastrophic-climate-change-202287

Barraclough, K. A., Carey, M., Winkel, K. D., Humphries, E., Shay, B. A., & Foong, Y. C. (2023). Why losing Australia's biodiversity matters for human health: Insights from the latest State of the Environment assessment. *Medical Journal of Australia*, 218(8), 336–340. https://doi.org/10.5694/mja2.51904

Climate Action Tracker. Available at: All countries. https://climateactiontracker.org/. Australia: https://climateactiontracker.org/countries/australia/

Climate Council. Available at: https://www.climatecouncil.org.au/

Combe, M., Evans, M. C., & Pelle, N. (2023). Losing the natural world comes with major risks for your super fund and bank. *The Conversation*, 3 February. https://theconversation.com/losing-the-natura l-world-comes-with-major-risks-for-your-super-fund-and-bank-198669

HEAL Network & CRE-STRIDE. (2021). Climate change and Aboriginal and Torres Strait Islander health. Discussion paper. Melbourne, Victoria: Lowitja Institute. https//doi.org/10.48455/bthg-aj15.

Myers, S., & Frumkin, H. (2020). *Planetary health. Protecting nature to protect ourselves*. Washington, DC: Island Press. https//doi.org/20.5822/978-1-61091-966-1

Romanello, M., Di Napoli, C., Drummond, P., Green, C., Kennard, H., *et al.* (2022). The 2022 report of the Lancet Countdown on health and climate change: Health at the mercy of fossil fuels. *Lancet*, 400 (10363), 1619–1654. https://doi.org/10.1016/S0140-6736(22)01540–9

References

Armistead, A., Campbell, R., Littleton, E., & Parrott, S. (2022). Fossil fuel subsidies in Australia. Federal and state government assistance to fossil fuel producers and major users in 2021–2022. Melbourne, Victoria: The Australian Institute. Available at: https://australiainstitute.org.au/wp-content/up loads/2022/03/P1198-Fossil-fuel-subsidies-2022-WEB.pdf (accessed 30 November 2022).

Australian Bureau of Statistics. (2022). Headline estimates of employment, unemployment, underemployment, participation and hours worked from the monthly Labour Force Survey. Reference period October 2022. Australian Government. https://www.abs.gov.au/statistics/labour/employment-a nd-unemployment/labour-force-australia/oct-2022(accessed 1 December 2022).

Australian Industry and Skills Committee. (n.d.). Coal mining. Available at: https://nationalindustryinsights. aisc.net.au/industries/mining-drilling-and-civil-infrastructure/coal-mining (accessed 1 December 2022).

Baade, P., Lu, C., Dasgupta, P., Cameron, J., & Fritschi, L. (2021). Prevalence of coal mine dust lung disease in Queensland, 1983/84–2019/20. Final Report. Queensland: Cancer Council Queensland. Available at: https://www.publications.qld.gov.au/ckan-publications-attachments-prod/resources/a78f60c0-dca7-4cca -b747-ec06fc926116/cmdld-prevalence-report.pdf?ETag=f5f239a85c76094c59d65a2b9af5421b

Baer, H. A. (2016). The nexus of the coal industry and the state in Australia: Historical dimensions and contemporary challenges. *Energy Policy*, 99, 194–202. https://doi.org/10.1016/j.enpol.2016.05.033

Cresswell, I., Janke, T., & Johnston, E. L. (2021). Australia, State of the Environment, 2021. Canberra: Commonwealth of Australia. Available at: https://soe.dcceew.gov.au

Crowley, K. (2021). Climate wars, carbon taxes and toppled leaders: The 30-year history of Australia's climate response, in brief. *The Conversation*. Available at: https://theconversation.com/climate-wars-carbon-taxes-and-toppled-leaders-the-30-year-history-of-australias-climate-response-in-brief-169545 (accessed 29 November 2022).

Ebi, K. L., Capon, A., Berry, P., Broderick, C., de Dear, R., Havenith, G., Honda, Y., Kovats, R. S., Ma, W., Malik, A., Morris, N. B., Nybo, L., Seneviratne, S. I., Vanos, J., & Jay, O. (2021). Hot weather and heat extremes: Health risks. *Lancet*, 398(10301), 698–708. https://doi.org/10.1016/S0140-6736(21)01208-3

Glavovic, B. C., Smith, T. F., & White, I. (2021). The tragedy of climate change science. *Climate and Development*, 14(9), 829–833. https://doi.org/10.1080/17565529.2021.2008855

IPBES. (2019). Summary for policymakers of the global assessment report on biodiversity and ecosystem services of the Intergovernmental Science-Policy Platform on Biodiversity and Ecosystem Services. IPBES Secretariat.

IPCC, Masson-Delmotte, V., Zhai, P., Pirani, A., Connors, S. L., Péan, C., Berger, S., Caud, N., Chen, Y., Goldfarb, L., Gomis, M. I., Huang, M., Leitzell, K., Lonnoy, E., Matthews, J. B. R., Maycock, T. K., Waterfield, T., … Zhou, B. (2021). Climate change 2021: The physical science basis. Contribution of Working Group I to the Sixth Assessment Report of the Intergovernmental Panel on Climate Change. Summary for policymakers. Available at: https://www.ipcc.ch/report/ar6/wg1/downloads/report/IPCC_AR6_WGI_SPM.pdf

Longden, T. (2019). The impact of temperature on mortality across different climate zones. *Climate Change*, 157(2), 221–242. https://doi.org/10.1007/s10584-019-02519-1

Millennium Ecosystem Assessment. (2005). *Ecosystems and human well-being: Synthesis*. Washington, DC: Island Press. Available at: https://www.millenniumassessment.org/documents/document.356.aspx.pdf

Myers, S. (2020). Food and nutrition on a rapidly changing planet. In S. Myers & H. Frumkin (Eds.), *Planetary health. Protecting nature to protect ourselves*. Washington, DC: Island Press. https://doi.org/https://doi.org/10.5822/978-1-61090-966-1

New South Wales Government. (n.d.) Regional NSW. Royalties. Available at: https://www.regional.nsw.gov.au/meg/community/royalties (accessed 1 December 2022).

Oreskes, N., & Conway, E. M. (2010). Defeating the merchants of doubt. *Nature*, 465(7299), 686–687. https://doi.org/10.1038/465686a

Oreskes, N., Conway, E., Karoly, D. J., Gergis, J., Neu, U., & Pfister, C. (2018). The denial of global warming. In *The Palgrave handbook of climate history*. London: Palgrave Macmillan, pp. 149–171. https://doi.org/10.1057/978-1-137-43020-5_14Polasky, S., & Dampha, N. K. (2021). Discounting and global environmental change. *Annual Review of Environment and Resources*, 46, 691–717. https://doi.org/10.1146/annurev-environ-020420-042100

Queensland Government. (2022). Budget strategy and outlook 2022–23, 4.4.3 Royalty Revenue. Available at: https://budget.qld.gov.au/files/Budget_2022-23_BP2_Revenue_Coal_Royalties.pdf (accessed 1 December 2022).

Safe Work Australia. (2012). Mining fact sheet 2011–12. Canberra: Commonwealth of Australia. Available at: https://www.safeworkaustralia.gov.au/system/files/documents/1702/mining-fact-sheet-2011-12.pdf (accessed 1 December 2022).

Statista. (2022). Number of employees in the oil and gas extraction industry in Australia from financial year 2012 to 2021. Available at: https://www.statista.com/statistics/692178/australia-employment-in-oil-and-gas-industry/(accessed 1 December 2022).

Stutzer, R., Rinscheid, A., Oliveira, T. D., Loureiro, P. M., Kachi, A., & Duygan, M. (2021). Black coal, thin ice: The discursive legitimisation of Australian coal in the age of climate change. *Humanities and Social Sciences*, 8(1). https://doi.org/10.1057/s41599-021-00827-5

Summers, J. K., & Smith, L. M. (2014). The role of social and intergenerational equity in making changes in human well-being sustainable. *Ambio*, 43(6), 718–728. https://doi.org/10.1007/s13280-013-0483-6

Supran, G., & Oreskes, N. (2017). Assessing ExxonMobil's climate change communications (1977–2014). *Environmental Research Letters*, 12(8), Article 084019. https://doi.org/10.1088/1748-9326/aa815f

Supran, G., & Oreskes, N. (2021). Rhetoric and frame analysis of ExxonMobil's climate change communications. *One Earth*, 4(5), 696–719. https://doi.org/10.1016/j.oneear.2021.04.014

Walter, C. M., Schneider-Futschik, E. K., Lansbury, N. L., Sly, P. D., Head, B. W., & Knibbs, L. D. (2021). The health impacts of ambient air pollution in Australia: a systematic literature review. *Internal Medicine Journal*, 51(10), 1567–1579. https://doi.org/10.1111/imj.15415

Wood, D., Griffiths, K., & Chivers, C. (2018). Who's in the room? Access and influence in Australian politics. Available at: https://grattan.edu.au/wp-content/uploads/2018/09/908-Who-s-in-the-room -Access-and-influence-in-Australian-politics.pdf

World Health Organization. (2010). A conceptual framework for action on the social determinants of health. Available at: https://apps.who.int/iris/handle/10665/44489

World Health Organization. (2021). WHO climate change and health factsheet, 2021. Available at: http s://www.who.int/news-room/fact-sheets/detail/climate-change-and-health

Index

Entries in **bold** denote tables; entries in *italics* denote figures.